# PERPETUALITY

# PERPETUALITY

## (A Perplexed Perpetual Reality with Illusions of Delusions)
## VOLUME 1

---

Allana Davis

(PERPETUALITY)
Copyright © 2020 by (Allana Shirelle Davis)

All rights reserved. No part of this book may be reproduced or transmitted in any form or by any means without written permission from the author.

ISBN: 978-0-578-23954-5

## Dedication

This book is dedicated to the women whose lives were taken by the hands of domestic violence, the women that did not make it out, the victims who did not survive. I am grateful, blessed, and fortunate to have lived; to be able to share my story; to help other victims who are still struggling with the decision to leave; and to shed some light for the victims' families and friends so they can know what domestic violence looks, feels, and sounds like.

*And no wonder, for even Satan disguises himself as an angel of light.*

2 Corinthians 11:14

# Contents

Introduction ............................................................. 1

Chapter One .......................................................... 2

Chapter Two .......................................................... 9

Chapter Three ..................................................... 28

Chapter Four ....................................................... 50

Chapter Five ........................................................ 67

Chapter Six .......................................................... 82

Chapter Seven ..................................................... 97

Chapter Eight .................................................... 119

Chapter Nine ..................................................... 148

Acknowledgments ............................................. 150

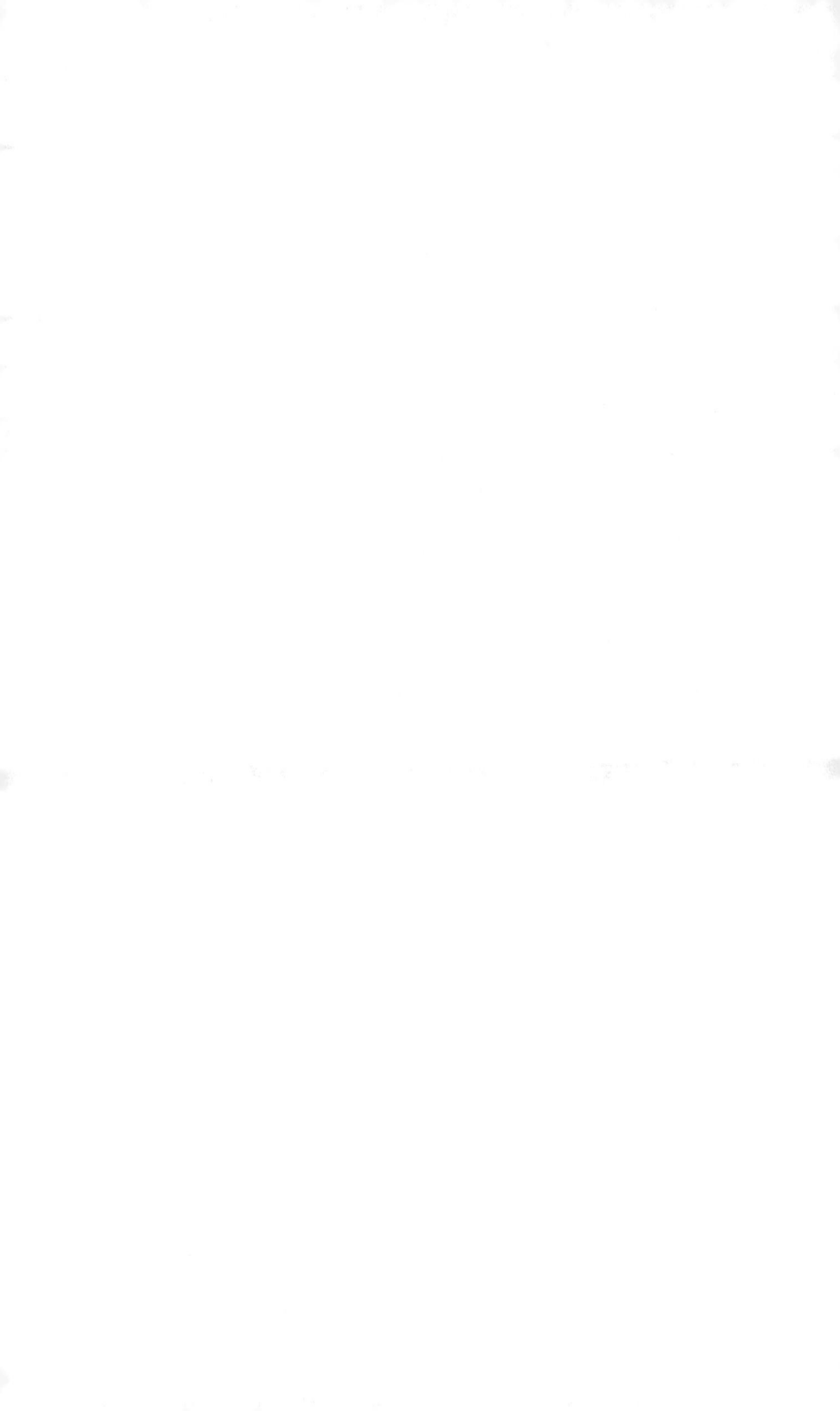

# Introduction

This book is about my experience with domestic violence. I want my readers to understand the details of what a woman really goes through behind closed doors; details of things that, most of the time, her family and friends have no clue about. I want my story to help women who are currently experiencing domestic violence to have the courage to leave. I'm sure it will also answer a lot of questions for victims and their families, or anyone who needs confirmation that they are in a toxic and abusive relationship, but still doubts themselves.

## Chapter One

"Lana, what the hell is going on? Why are you in jail? Where is Raymond?"

High school sweethearts—that's what I thought we were in the beginning. I would always notice—and you couldn't help but notice—this young, brown-skinned man of medium build, about five foot nine, with a very infectious smile and a personality that changed the atmosphere. When he walked in he was loud and boisterous. That's why I noticed him or paid him any attention, as he walked behind my register as I was itemizing my customer's purchase.

"Who the hell is this, talking all loud?" I said to myself. I tried not to look at him. I did my best to focus and really act like I was concentrating on the order. I was praying that my nervousness wasn't showing.

"How are you doing?" he asked.

"Fine, how are you?"

"I'm good. Thanks for asking. How do you say your name? All-*ah*-na?"

"No, it's All-*a*-na. The second 'A' is long," I said, correcting him with a grin.

"Oh, I'm sorry Allana."

"That's okay."

"I'm Golden."

"Oh, Golden," I said, grinning from ear to ear.

"You have a very pretty smile," he said flirtatiously.

"Thank you."

"What time you get off?"

"In about half an hour, 7:30."

I was seventeen when I met him at Wegmans, a grocery store where we both worked. I was a cashier and he worked in the helping hands department, pushing carts and assisting customers load their groceries into their vehicles. He came through my line one day with one item, a sixteen-ounce Sprite. The customer before him had over 300 dollars' worth of groceries, and on top of that, there were too many express lines open. I knew something was up. And what do you know—after introducing himself, he asked if he could meet me outside when I clocked out. I was so shy when I talked to him. I gave him my phone number and he gave me his on a piece of paper, with the name Golden written on it. I felt like I was on top of the world then. I had this five foot nine, light-skinned man named Golden, with big, luscious lips and a bright smile, asking for my phone number.

I had just gotten out of another relationship a few months prior, it was my junior year, and my prom was around the corner. I thought meeting Golden was right on time. I came to find out he was in a program called "Life's Choices" at Monroe Community College in downtown Rochester, New York, where I was getting tutoring for a Geometry course I was taking at East High School. He would come to see me at the times he knew I was getting tutored.

After one of my tutoring sessions, Golden came to see me as usual. As he sat across from me at the table smiling, he said, "What the hell is that on your cheek?"

I was so fucking embarrassed. "It's a pimple," I said in a calm, hesitant voice.

"That's a goddamn zit," he said, laughing out loud. I laughed along with him as if he hadn't hurt my feelings.

Within the first two months of talking to Raymond, which was Golden's real name, he asked me to be his girlfriend. I said yes. We left around the same time for different trips around spring break. He was going on a Black College trip with a group from Monroe Community College (MCC). He gave me his information, his agenda, rather, so I could get in touch with him. That made me feel really good, like I could trust him.

I was on honor roll, and my grades got me into the Jasco program, which would prepare me to receive a scholarship for college. As one of the top three students, I was chosen to go on the Black College Tour for free. All I had to bring was spending money.

Out of all the colleges I visited down south from state to state, I wanted to attend Clark Atlanta University in Atlanta, Georgia. (I absolutely love Atlanta, where I sit right now as I write my story. I'm in my favorite spot at the Underground, in front of the waterfalls.)

When I arrived back home from the Black College tour and got back to school, I heard through a classmate that went on the same college tour as Raymond that he had been dealing with another female. It was his ex-girlfriend, Shauna. She said that they had been kissing and hugging on the roller coaster at Busch Gardens, and even had sex.

I confronted him about the issue over the telephone. He said they had just talked and that they got in an argument. Of course, I believed him. He said I couldn't believe rumors from other people. He said it was all lies.

I remember inviting a good friend from Chicago, Chris, to go to church with me. Chris worked at the same grocery store. After church, I was afraid because Raymond was there too. I wanted to invite my friend Chris over for dinner, like my mom asked me to, but feeling intimidated by Raymond, I completely cut Chris short, and I knew I had offended him. I never saw or talked to Chris again.

That was just of one of many red flags I had already experienced within just a few months of dating Raymond. He had made it clear that he was the only man that I was to give my attention to.

\* \* \*

As Raymond yelled my name up the stairs of my house, I got an awkward feeling and the atmosphere became uncomfortable. I felt out of place, and I could hear all my family in the house asking, "Why is he yelling her name like that?"

"Let's go, Lana!" he yelled in a rushing and controlling voice. Like I had to hurry up, or else.

He had rented a white compact car for us, and my two male friends from church, my sister, and my cousin were supposed to follow us. We were going to Darien Lake for Grand Nite. For junior and seniors from local area high schools, the amusement park opened late, from 12 a.m. until about 7 a.m. I don't remember saying much of anything in the car. I remember him doing a whole lot of speeding, asking him to slow down, and being on pins and needles. I was unhappy that night, and so uncomfortable. As much as I loved Darien Lake, I had such a horrible time, especially after he got an attitude and walked off. I ended up going home with my sister, cousin, and two male friends. More red flags appeared, and I just ignored them. Month after month, year after year, it would continue to get worse.

On my junior prom night, Raymond tried to have sex with me. I liked the hugging, kissing, and touching, but I didn't have sex with him. I was a virgin. He didn't believe I was, because most of the girls or young women my age already had kids.

It wasn't long until I did have sex with him, about seven months into the relationship. One night after I got off work, he took me to his place where he lived with his grandparents, Mr. and Mrs. Perry. He picked me up and carried me up the stairs so we wouldn't wake them up. He lit a candle and played some slow music. I was turned on, but scared at the same time. He was making me feel so damn good. I was comfortable. Then he said, "Just let me stick the head in." I let him, of course, and after that it was a wrap, I was open. We told each other I love you, and yes, I felt like I was in heaven on earth, when he went down and made love to me with his big-ass juicy lips. I was hooked.

My grades dropped tremendously. I started skipping a majority of my classes and hanging out pass curfew, sometimes not coming home until the next day. On one occasion, my mom called his grandparents' house to see where I was. We had my mom's car that night, and I was still out after two or three in the morning. We were in the part of the basement Raymond had fixed up as his bedroom. Mr. Perry, his grandfather, called Raymond on his cell phone to see where we were. Even though we were right downstairs in the basement, he lied and said that we had just picked up my Aunt Charmaine from the Amtrak train station and dropped her off at home. I couldn't sneak out and leave until they went to bed.

Eventually, Raymond got his own apartment, and after I barely graduated high school, I moved in with him. My mother was furious. If it hadn't been for the Lord Jesus Christ, my mother, and summer school, I would not have graduated high school. I had already encountered mental, verbal, and emotional abuse. In spite of it all, I still stayed with Raymond and thought I was in love.

We got into an argument, I don't remember what about. He threw me on the bed and held me down tight with his hands around my wrists. I believe he got mad because I had talked back to him, and he didn't like it. My brother Andre was in the other room. I didn't want him to know what was going on, so I kept quiet. It hurt like hell, especially when I saw his fingerprints on my skin. I thought I was wrong and to blame for his behavior.

I tried to hide the fingerprints, but my mother noticed one evening when I went to her house. I think I had forgotten all about them. She said I better not let my stepdad, Melvin, or my dad, William, find out Raymond's putting his hands on me. That's if I didn't want any trouble.

No matter what my mother or anybody else said, I continued to stay with him. She encouraged me to get out of the relationship. She knew it wasn't good, but I wasn't listening.

\* \* \*

My first suspicion that Raymond was cheating on me was when he was living with his grandparents. I went downstairs in the basement to his bedroom, and he had an 8x10 picture of his ex-girlfriend Shauna—not my picture. My feeling was that he'd had her in his room sometime before I got there. I didn't say anything at first, because deep down I knew he was going to give me an excuse. I don't even remember what it was he said, but I accepted it. My self-esteem had already vanished. I had none.

While I was there, he would put the cordless phone by him, answer it, get up, and walk out the door. I knew he was going to see Shauna around the corner. This happened on plenty of occasions. Later down the line, I started finding condoms, pictures, and phone numbers of other women. I left him, but kept going back for more pain.

I remember having to go to the clinic one day because something was just not right with me. I was having a nasty discharge. I found out that I had trichomoniasis, a sexually transmitted disease (STD). I don't remember what excuse Raymond had for that. Shauna was calling more frequently and hanging up the phone when I answered. One day, she left a message that she had gone to the doctor and had been diagnosed for the same STD.

Shauna and I talked on a couple of occasions. She told me things about how he'd been with her and when. She was able to repeat conversations that Raymond and I had—things I know she couldn't have made up. At the time, Shauna and I attended the same college. We were going to approach Raymond about his cheating when he came to pick me up from school. Somehow, he found out. I'm sure she told him, because I sure as hell didn't. He never picked me up from school. I was naïve, because for all I know she could've set me up and tried to get me jumped. Shauna and I caught the RTS bus together, and still wanted to confront him at his apartment when I got home. But he was nowhere in sight.

Eventually his relationship with Shauna faded out, but matters still grew worse. At this first apartment, a neighbor called the cops because we got into a physical and bloody argument. Neither of us went to jail. After it happened, I left and went to my mom's house. This was during the same time that we decided to go to Frederick Douglass Football Field at two o'clock in the morning, and called ourselves making love in the rain. We lathered each other with Ivory Soap and started making out on the field. The moment was ruined when my coochie started burning from the soap.

## Chapter Two

One of my most embarrassing moments was in 1998, when we went to Freaknik in Atlanta. We stayed with Raymond's cousins in Stone Mountain. They didn't even know we were coming. It was a surprise, but they were happy to see us.

Around the same time, I noticed the financial abuse when he asked me to sign up for a Kaufman's charge card to pay for Nautica sports jackets for both of us. Each one was $150, and we never paid off the charge card. I didn't feel good about myself at all. I didn't feel good-looking. I felt stupid and dumb, like he said I was. I felt even worse when he was flirting with the women, recording them with his camcorder and taking pictures of them, making disrespectful comments out loud in front of me. Then, I was left at his cousins' house all night long until he came back at five or six in the morning. They didn't like how I was being treated.

One night, Raymond, his cousin, and I all decided to go to Club 112, which was located on Lavista Road in the plaza. We got in line to go inside the nightclub. He cussed me out and called me names out loud in public because I didn't wear a certain outfit—short, skin-tight, or see-through. I didn't look like the rest of the women that he was looking at. When we finally got to the entrance, we found out that I couldn't get in. I had to be twenty-one years old to get in, but I was only twenty. He got pissed off, got an attitude with me, and started yelling at me. As I walked away from him, he started walking towards me as if he was going to hit me. His cousin warned him not to do it, because that was one thing the police did not tolerate, and then he would be in jail. He turned back around and went in the club, and that was another night I didn't see him until later the next morning.

*Perpetuality*

We got into it one of these mornings while his older cousin Meechie was at home. Meechie was such a sweet lady. She heard us tussling, and when I started screaming, Meechie yelled at us to break up our fighting. Her blood pressure ran high because he had badmouthed her, too. She was surprised. This fight got back to Raymond's grandmother, Mrs. Perry, because she and his cousins were related, and then back to my mother and the rest of the family.

When Meechie and I had a chance to be alone, she was lying on the bed trying to calm down. She said, "I know he's your first love and you love him, but he doesn't deserve you. He's not the one for you." As bad as he had acted towards Meechie and I, I heard what she said, but I didn't want to hear it. I knew she was telling the truth, but I still wanted to hope that he would change.

Around this time and before the trip, I had noticed phone numbers of different women in his cell phone. One particular woman's number I noticed during the trip. He was outside, talking on the cordless phone. I picked up the receiver carefully in the bedroom I was in, and it was her on the other end. I listened. It was flirtatious talk, and it sounded like they were into each other. I hung up the phone carefully and didn't say anything. If I recall correctly, she sent him some money.

We ended up staying in Atlanta with his cousins for two weeks, one week more than we were supposed to, and the car we'd rented was in his friend Mike's name. Raymond got a phone call from Mike to hurry back home to Rochester, because he was going to have to pay for this extra week he wasn't expecting to pay for, and on top of that, he had been fired from his job. I lost count of how many jobs he'd had, including one at Xerox. He always was able to get well-paying jobs, but couldn't keep them.

When we got back home from Atlanta, Raymond commanded me to call in to work to ask for hours. The same day we got back I started working, because he told me to. I was working as a home health aide at the time, and I was on a per-diem schedule, so I could basically make my own hours. By 1999, we had already moved into our fourth apartment. I had gotten my certification to be a Certified Nursing Assistant in the early spring of that year, and I got hired permanently full-time at The Friendly Home, where I was trained.

On top of the stress from the relationship, I was the only one working steady. I had to work the 3-11 p.m. shift because that's what they offered me, even though I preferred the day shift. I started to deal with more dishonesty and disrespect with Raymond. I started noticing that some of my clothes and items went missing at times. I had found a women's earring in my bed, and I knew it wasn't mine. On one occasion, I remember looking on top of the entertainment center and noticed my junior prom picture with Raymond was missing. I knew he hid it because he'd had another female in the house. I searched and searched, and finally, what do you know, there it was—placed under the cushion of the couch. I felt rage come over me. I felt numb at the same time, like, *how in the hell could this happen?*

Late night while he was out, I received a phone call from a female. She threatened me that she was coming to my house to do something, kick my motherfucking ass, this that and the other.

"Bitch, I wish you would!" I told her. No one ever came. Of course, when I approached him, he didn't know who it was. He started staying out later and later. Six a.m. turned into ten and eleven a.m. His reason was that he had fallen asleep at his man or cousin's house. I remember staying up all night, pacing the floor, calling his grandmother's house, or whoever's place I knew he was supposed to be at, and they hadn't seen him. I was calling all the area hospitals and jails, and they didn't have anybody by his name.

*Perpetuality*

One morning, I was getting off an overnight shift of 11 p.m.–7 a.m. As I walked up the driveway, I noticed a black Ford. I felt my stomach on fire as I got closer. I went to open the screen door, and it was locked. I couldn't use my key to get in the house. My curiosity grew more and more. I yelled, "Raymond, Raymond, open the door!" I banged as hard as I could. I went to the back door, but the chain was on the door. I knew he had someone in the house.

As I returned to the front, I tried to get through the bedroom window. He said, "I'm coming." He made it sound like I was crazy for wanting to get in my own house. After a good fifteen or more minutes, by the time he let me in, I could tell he had been asleep, and that he had snuck the person out. Whoever she was, I didn't get to see what she looked like.

I asked, "What the hell took you so long to open the door?"

He said that he had been sleeping hard, and he didn't hear me. I noticed an empty bottle of E&J. I asked him about the leather coat and keys.

"That's Isaac's coat and keys," he said. "He drove Kesha's car last night, but the car wouldn't start."

What a fat-ass lie. First of all, I knew that wasn't Isaac's coat, because he wasn't that big, and Kesha drove a white jeep. I never saw her drive this black Ford. He rushed out of the house with the coat and keys in his hand, stating he was going to drop them off to Isaac. He was avoiding me asking him more questions. He knew I was on to him.

On another day, I started getting that burning feeling in my stomach again as I was on the RTS bus, getting closer to the house. A while ago, I remembered seeing this teal Ford compact car while Raymond and I were out taking a stroll in the area where we lived. I noticed it from about twenty feet away. Inside was a dark-skinned chick, and she honked the horn as she slowed down, looking our way.

"Golden!" she yelled. I never called him by his nickname. He looked up with a frown on his face, as if he didn't know who it was. He walked over to the car, and conversed for about two minutes. I was scared to go over there with him, so I stayed where I was until he came back. I felt like a fool; I felt stupid. I felt like I was in a dark tunnel, and it was a bright sunny day. I knew something wasn't right. I didn't say anything when he came back over. I didn't want to start an argument. I didn't want him to think I didn't trust him, like he had told me many times before. Finally, about twenty minutes later, I asked, "Who was that?"

"Why you wait so long to ask me?"

"I don't know. Who was she?"

"That was my cousin."

"Your cousin. I have never seen or met her before."

"If you don't believe me, you can ask my grandmother. She's my cousin on my father's side of the family. Her name is Tammy. You don't remember meeting her before?"

"No, I don't. I'm sure I would've remembered."

"I'm sorry, I thought you met her."

I left it alone and didn't say anything else about it.

One night, when I saw the same teal car at our place after coming home from work, my first thought was, *Why would his cousin be here after 11:30 at night by herself? Or maybe she didn't come by herself.* As I put my key in the door and stepped in the apartment, I saw her in a pivot position on the couch, where his feet were, as he lied there with his shirt open. The television was playing Jerry Springer, and there were no lights on. Neither one of them heard me come into the apartment. I wasn't even standing five feet away. I could have killed them both. I threw the glass lamp on the floor. They woke up in disbelief, as if they were both shocked they had lost track of time.

*Perpetuality*

"What the hell is going on?" I screamed. "You call this bitch your cousin?" I punched, scratched, and slapped him. He was trying to stop me from going after her as she rushed out the door. I was mad and pissed off at myself for not locking her in the house when I had the chance, so I could jump and beat her like no tomorrow. As I had a chance to think, I remembered the name McKenzie coming up on our caller ID at our last apartment, when we stayed under his mother. I realized it was her calling way back then, some months back. We didn't stay in any apartment long. I don't remember staying in one for even a solid year.

One night, Raymond thought I was sound asleep. It was about four o'clock in the morning. Most nights I would sleep hard because I was that tired. I was fully awake, but I made him believe otherwise. He smelled real funky to me, because he was supposed to be at work, and didn't get off until six in the morning. I could hear him going down into the basement. I knew he kept colored condoms in the top drawer. I began to sweat, and then became cold, as I saw him take one or two from the bag. He still thought I was asleep.

I gave him five minutes so I could run and bust him out. Then, I ran as fast as I could down the basement stairs. I saw him standing up by Scandalous, our pit bull dog, who was in her cage. Come to think of it, I almost went to jail one night because Scandalous had gotten sick. The Rochester Police tracked me down at my mom and stepdad's house while they were celebrating their anniversary in the Poconos. My Aunt Charmaine answered the door. I was going to go to jail by midnight because a check that I wrote had bounced, and they were coming back for me if I didn't pay the debt to the veterinarian in Pittsford.

In the basement, Raymond was barefoot.

"What are you doing?" I asked.

"Nothing," he said, looking like Scandalous the pit bull when she knows she's fucked up. He was breathing hard, and he was trying to control it, but it wasn't working. As I walked closer to him, I saw a woman. She was dark-skinned. No, this was not the one he said was his cousin. She was on the heavy side. She sat on the basement floor, butt naked, with just her white and green striped shirt on. When she looked up at me, she looked as if she had glue on her face. I had called on Jesus before I ran down into this situation, and he was with me. I just stood there and said, "Hi."

"Hi," she said with a half-smile. "Oh my God," she then said in an embarrassed tone as she turned her face.

"Boo, it's not what you think. See, what happened—her and her man got in an argument at the gas station, he tried to rape her, and she was running away from the gas station half-naked. She asked me to help her. Could you see if I have a pair of extra jogging pants in the drawer?"

I kept calm the whole time. I wanted to bust out laughing. She went right along with the story. She said her boyfriend kicked her out of the car, and that it was a blue Neon.

"What?!" I said, as if I was concerned. I said okay, walked back upstairs, grabbed the phone, and called the police.

"911, what's your emergency?"

"Yes, my name is Allana Parrish, and I have a half-naked woman in my basement that's saying she had been arguing with her boyfriend and that he almost raped her, but she got away. I am calling from 355 North Goodman Street."

"The officer is on his way, Miss Parrish."

"Thank you."

I anxiously waited for the police to arrive while they both were still downstairs, thinking I was looking for jogging pants. Within five minutes the police came. I waved them down while I stood in the driveway. There were two policemen. One drove up right after the other.

"What's going on here?" the officer asked.

"Well, there's a half-naked woman in my basement that said she was almost raped."

"Are you the one that called us?"

"Yes, sir."

"And what's your name?"

"Allana Parrish."

I walked them towards the basement, and I came down the stairs first. I looked at their faces carefully, and both of their looks were unexplainable, especially when they saw the police come down behind me.

"Ma'am, we understand that you almost got raped."

"Yes, officer."

As they listened to her made-up story, I noticed an empty condom wrapper on the floor. As they both tried to get the police to believe their story, I stayed quiet and just observed. I looked at Officer Conan's face, and I could tell he thought something was fishy about the situation. His partner asked, "Allana, do you have a towel or sheet or something?"

"Sure."

"Ma'am, are you hurt? Do you need to go to the hospital?"

I came back down and gave her a sheet. She gave the officer her name and said she lived out in the country, Wayne County, with her mother and some friends. She was on her cell phone calling for a ride, as she made it seem. I don't remember how she got home till this day. I didn't give her any pants to put on, maybe Raymond did. It was about

6:30 a.m. by the time the cops left. I could tell by their faces they were going to have a ball laughing about this particular call.

After, I went to the gas station right across the street, where they said the incident happened. I knew it all was a lie, but I had to ask the attendant anyway to make myself feel better.

"Good morning. Could you tell me if you saw a couple arguing and fighting in a blue Neon, or a half-naked lady get kicked out of the car about an hour ago?"

He shook his head and said no.

"You didn't see anything?"

"No, I've been here all night."

"Thank you."

As I turned and walked away, I felt empty, even though I had the confirmation that it was a lie. I didn't know if I was coming or going. I felt like I had nothing to live for.

Later on that day, my mom asked me to go with her to do some running around. I felt like she had saved me from a burning fire. I was anxious to go. I needed to get away.

As my mother was getting in the car, the words from a Kurt Carr gospel song came on. "*God's mercy kept me so I wouldn't let go. I almost let go. I felt like I just couldn't take life anymore. My problems had me bound. Depression weighed me down, but God held me close. So I wouldn't let go.*" The words just made me break. I cried out loud in such agony with my face in my hands. My mom reached over and held me tight. "It's going to be okay," she said. Even at this moment, I can still feel her hugging me tight. I felt safe in her arms, like I was going to be okay.

"Oh my God Lana, what's wrong? Talk to me."

"I found him in the basement with another girl."

"What?" my mom said in a shocked voice. "Baby, I can't make your decisions for you. You're grown now. All I can do is talk to you.

*Perpetuality*

You don't deserve this. When are you going to get enough? Do you want to come home?" she said softly.

"Yes."

I went the next day to pack and get my stuff to go stay with my mom. Of course, you know I still went back. This wasn't the only time I had left.

One night at the same apartment on Goodman Street, I had my mother take me to get my winter coat that I had left. That teal Ford was in the driveway. This was at night.

"Whose car is that?" my mom asked.

"Oh, that's his cousin," I said quickly. I knew Tammy was in there, and she sure as hell wasn't his cousin. I didn't want to tell my mom everything. I knocked and banged, and even tried to open the bedroom window, but I couldn't get in. My mom was getting pissed off at the situation.

"Do you want me to call the police? He's in there, but not coming to the door," she said as she blew the car horn over and over. I gave her the okay to call the police. The police came and they couldn't get in. Even then, no one came to the door. I believe they were hiding. I left it alone and went back another time. When we got back together sometime after that, he said Tammy came over that night because she came to his rescue when he told her he was going to commit suicide.

"Golden, please don't do it," she said, and she rushed over to the house. Raymond said they were hiding and he was scared. He didn't want any drama. *Excuses, excuses, excuses*, I thought. We were on our way to move out in the suburbs, Greece, New York, out of the city. His grandmother Mrs. Perry had bought him a Honda Accord for $2,000, and he sold it for $4,500. It was a '91 or '92. He got the interior painted a little bit, sky blue, like the outside. It was cute. When he first brought the car home, I was disappointed, because it was a stick shift. I didn't how to drive one really well. The first time I drove a stick was when his grandmother co-signed a Plymouth Breeze for him, when we stayed at our first apartment. He taught me here and there. One night, I was put in a situation to drive his car because he went to jail for stealing and using somebody else's credit card. The cops chased him from Irondequoit Mall. They caught him hiding in an auto shop garage, where the owner pointed him out. I was the only one he could count on that night to get the car, or it would be towed. I had to remember how to shift the gears. It was very frustrating, but I learned and got the car back safely to the apartment.

 He sold the Honda so we could get furniture for the townhouse we were moving into. It was a white man and his 17- year old daughter, who looked like she was mixed, that bought the car. We were still living at the apartment on Goodman Street when they saw the car for sale. The girl fell in love with it when she looked inside and saw the blue interior, and even more when she took it for a test drive. The father paid Raymond $4,500 in cash the very next week at our new place, which was the townhouse in Greece. That weekend we went to Value City to get cream Italian leather couches and glass tables, bought a 56" inch screen television from Rent-A-Center for $500, an entertainment center from Circuit City, a futon and 29" inch television for the finished basement, a 19" inch television for the guest room, a washer and dryer, and odds and ends for the rest of the house. The townhouse was lovely, but I felt like I wasn't there. I still felt alone and unhappy most of the time.

 I had started working at Monroe Community Hospital around this time, rotating days and nights full-time. The benefits were lovely. I was the only one working most of the time, trying to pay rent, utilities, and other things. I noticed certain things going on. I knew how Raymond prepared dinner, but sometimes it was done differently. He was

*Perpetuality*

continually staying out all night. I was calling the hospitals and jails again. He would tell me more and more that I needed to start wearing my clothes a certain way, to have a provocative, promiscuous look. I had started buying a few outfits just like that. I noticed he was starting to drink more alcohol. I had a feeling that he and Tammy had something going on, and they were becoming serious, but I couldn't prove it.

I came home one morning from a night shift and he was supposed to be home. There was a blanket and pillow on the couch, as if he had been sleeping, but I also found open condom wrappers on the table, along with empty beer bottles and smoked cherry tips.

He had told me that Tammy had been having some trouble at home with her Mom, and she wasn't going to have anywhere to stay. For all I know, as he was talking to her on the phone that night, he made it sound like she was in a crisis. I told Raymond it was okay for her to come. She stayed with us for almost two weeks. By this time, she had apologized for the time on Goodman Street, that night I had caught them on the couch together, and said Raymond was like a big brother to her, and he had said the same thing. So they would hang out at times, go off like they were just brother and sister, and I accepted it like a fool. I even went to visit her church with her and sat with her. I held no grudges. I put the past in the past, but I found out I couldn't trust everybody that testifies, dances, and shouts, and Tammy did all of the above this same Sunday I went with her.

One night that next week, when I came home, Raymond said that she had moved out. I felt something was strange for her to just up and leave without saying anything.

"Hey Boo, this girl is tripping. She was starting to say that she thought we was both feeling each other, and she thought we were going to be together."

"Why would she think that?"

"Boo, I don't know. I was just trying to be nice."

The phone rang. "Hello?"

"Hi, Allana," she said hesitantly. "This is Tammy. We really need to talk. I'm woman enough and I think you should be woman enough."

Raymond was making it seem like it was all her, and she just turned on him. He sat on the couch, and after I hung up the phone, I was ready. I took my gold cross necklace and earrings off. I had on my sneakers and tank top, and started pacing the floor. I knew already that they had been lying. I was thinking, *she has the nerve to come to my house and start some shit, even though she said she just wanted to talk*? I had nothing to talk about.

*Ding Dong*, the doorbell rang.

Raymond answered the door. Tammy walked in and sat on the couch next to me.

"I just want to let the truth out," she said.

"Did you fuck him?" I asked.

"Yep," she said boldly.

All I remember is jumping on her and punching her with my fists. Raymond grabbed me off of her, but I scratched, kicked, and yelled, and told him to let me go. He was trying to keep us apart, but I got a hold of her by her micro-braids, and all I could feel was my adrenaline rushing, and I pinned her down on the other couch, punching on her. I noticed she started to dig her nails in my forearm, and I still didn't let go right away. He finally was able to pull me off, and the pain was starting to get to me. She stood up to take her jacket off and wanted to fight some more. She took my aromatherapy candle and threw it at me. I dodged it, and it put a hole in the wall. He was still trying to keep us apart. They both ran together in the kitchen and hid behind the wall, and I tried to hit them with the wine cooler, but I missed.

"That's enough! Y'all want to fight, y'all take it outside and fight," Raymond yelled as he opened the door.

"I'm not going to jail and getting kicked out for this bitch," I said as I dialed 911.

She ran down the bottom step, caught me off guard and smacked me in the face.

"You lied, you are a liar. You said that you were going to kick her out, and me and you was going to be together!" Tammy yelled.

"I'm not going no goddamn where, this is my house."

"Stop lying, this is Golden's house, and I'm not talking to you."

I started to get flushed. I wanted to do something real terrible to the both of them.

"Golden, who do you want to be with? Is it going to be me or her?"

"Tammy, Allana is the one I want to be with. You have to leave, please leave."

Tammy slapped his ass across the face. She ran upstairs looking like she had to throw up. By the time she came back downstairs, the police were at the door.

"What's the problem?" the officer asked.

"We just had a little fight," Raymond told the officer.

"Anybody hurt?"

"No officer."

"Who lives here?"

"We do," Raymond answered back like he's so innocent.

"Ma'am, I'm going to have to ask you to leave."

A couple of days later she apologized over the phone. I forgave her.

About two weeks later we went to Atlanta. Raymond got his best friend Mike to rent an Intrepid for him. I honestly don't remember anything good about this trip. We stayed at Raymond's cousin's house, whom we stayed with last time we were in Atlanta. We went to go look at some apartment complexes. We were talking about relocating then. I remember him getting mad at me, because I had my ID to look at the apartment and he had forgotten his. Since his older cousin who was in his 50s came with us, he looked at the apartment with me, along with the leasing agent. After cussing me out and throwing a tantrum, Raymond took off and left me with his cousins again. He felt disrespected because I decided to see the apartment without him. His cousins hadn't known me for long, but I heard at one time from Mrs. Perry, his grandmother, that they wondered what in the world I was doing with him. We stayed longer than planned, and when we did leave, it was because his friend told him a warrant was going to be put out to get the car back.

We needed money to get back home. Raymond pawned a gold chain that Tammy had bought him. He didn't get much for it. He called Tammy to send some money through Western Union. Yes, for us to get back home to Rochester. I got mad at him and spoke my mind about it. He said I should be glad, and that if it wasn't for her, we wouldn't be able to get home. We left Atlanta as soon as she sent the money, so we could get the car back.

"What's wrong? Why are you so quiet?"

"Nothing." I wanted to cry. I kept quiet the whole 15-16 hour trip back home. I don't remember what day of the week it was when we got back home, but my Aunt Charmaine called me days later to invite me to her church. I was hesitant because I knew I was living the wrong way. I had no business shacking up in the first place. I had always believed, and had it programmed in my mind, that you should live with and get to know the person before you get married, but as I write

*Perpetuality*

at this moment, I knew that was bologna. What God puts together is good, what he doesn't is not.

This particular Sunday, I was scheduled to go to work from 3-11 p.m. My Aunt gave me a ride. Come to find out when I got to the church, she had invited my mother, brothers, and sister also. My heart was rebellious at the time. I didn't want to hear the truth. I kept watching the clock, as I wished I could've gotten into my own car and just driven off. I ended up being late for work. When they did the alter call, God had a word for me. Aunt Charmaine stood by me and laid hands on me as the prophet gave me the word.

"You're planning a trip to relocate. Don't go. You also have some clothes in your closet that you need to get rid of. The man that you're with now, he's not for you. Your husband is going to be a man of God and you'll want for nothing."

I heard what he said, but didn't listen to him, at least not to everything. I did throw away the provocative clothes I had in my closet, and I didn't relocate to Atlanta at that time.

My mom Vanessa and Aunt Charmaine prayed me out of that townhouse. Three days later, I called them to come pick me up, and my luggage, so I could move back home with my mom. Raymond wasn't home when I left. I hadn't heard from him in about a week or two. When I did talk to him, he was telling me how serious he was about getting married. I still wanted to believe that things would get better between us, especially that if I became his wife, he would change. We made plans from there on, about five months away on July 15, 2000. This was the second time we set a date. The first time was a year before.

One night, we went to a revival at his mother's church. It was apostolic, the church of Jesus Christ. They held the revival that whole week. I had already gotten saved about nine years prior at my home church, which was Church of God in Christ (C.O.G.I.C), but had backslid. The second night I went, they called everyone who wanted to get filled with the Holy Ghost to come to the tarry room.

"Call him! Call him daughter! Call him! Say thank you Jesus, thank you Jesus, thaaaank ya!" A few of the church mothers yelled as they kneeled down beside me, clapping and praying.

I wanted to say, "Would ya'll stop yelling and spitting on me? Please."

"Thank you Jesus. Thank you Jesus. Jesus, Jesus, Jesus, Je...Je...Je...Je...Je...Je...Je...Je...Je...Je...Jesus."

I started drooling and slobbering at the mouth. I just let it go.

"She got it! Hallelujah, she got filled with the Holy Ghost," Raymond's mother, Evangelist Chapman yelled.

A couple of nights later, he said he'd been filled with the Holy Ghost too. We celebrated. The ministers at this church encouraged me to get baptized in Jesus' name because the C.O.G.I.C. way was wrong, so I did. Raymond said he'd already gotten baptized when he was younger. After that, I guess they considered me as a member, or going to be, but I already had a church home. The ministers encouraged us to go and get married. They had people at the Church of Jesus Christ who would do the flowers, make the dresses, and so forth. They said only saved people from that church could be allowed in our wedding. If my father wasn't saved, he could not walk me down the aisle. If my sister wasn't saved, she could not be my maid of honor, and so forth. We also couldn't get married with wedding rings. We had to buy and get married with watches.

Speaking of rings, Raymond hadn't given me a ring yet. During the five months of planning the wedding, it became frustrating to the very end. Since we knew we were getting married, we moved back into the city in a one bedroom not too far from my mother, on Rocket

*Perpetuality*

Street. My mom was excited to be helping with everything, but she didn't approve of who I was marrying. Neither did my Aunt, and a lot of others, including some of his family members. My family paid for the whole wedding, everything. Raymond hadn't paid for anything. He didn't have a job. I know, call me sick in the head.

*Allana Davis*

## BETTER FOR ME

Better for me to live than die. Better for me to sing than cry. Better for me to be free, than to live in bondage to a man who did not bleed and die for me. Better for me to run than stay, at least I won't be locked up in a cell or six feet deep, anyway. It's better for me now, because I got away. Nothing but God's grace and mercy, that I can say, I'm able to live again. Better for me.

National Domestic Violence Hotline: 1-800-799-7233

Maybe you are still in denial or disbelief, or still doubting yourself. STOP IT! H.E.E.D. THE RED FLAGS! (HATE+ ENVY + ENMITY + DENIAL & DISORIENTATION = DEATH)

# Chapter Three

I had noticed something in Raymond's notebook. It was odd to me, and I couldn't figure it out. It was his handwriting and somebody else's. They were conversing back and forth on the paper, and asking questions. Some of the conversation was sexual. I asked him about it, and he said that he was just playing a joke on me. He and one of his boys were writing to play a trick on me. He said, "What other reason would I leave it there for you to see it?" I accepted what he said and went on.

I called myself being open and honest about a picture I had taken with a Chippendale. The man had grabbed one of my breasts as the photographer snapped the picture. My sister and best friend took me to see the Chippendales before my wedding as a bachelorette party. I felt like I should've been honest about something like that. So I told him and showed him the picture. He accused me of cheating, called me all kinds of bitches and motherfuckers, threw me on the couch and started choking me. Later he said he was sorry, and asked if there was anything else I needed to tell him.

Down to the wire, it was getting closer to July 15th. I didn't get my ring until the week or two before, and when he gave it to me, he wasn't real. It wasn't the way I expected him to do it. No feeling or passion at all. The night before the wedding he went to a bachelor party his friends threw for him. I didn't feel confident about him going. He borrowed my Uncle D's Jeep Cherokee that night. We weren't supposed to see each other the night before the wedding, so I stayed at my mom's house, where Uncle D stayed at the time. Raymond got back to my mom's house about five o'clock in the morning, woke me up, and said that he had been in an accident with Uncle D's truck.

Raymond was drunk and could hardly talk straight. He said it wasn't his fault and that the car in front of him backed into the front bumper. The bumper was partially off. He told my Uncle that he would pay for it to be fixed. Uncle D never saw a penny. After that, Raymond went back to our apartment. I could hardly sleep. Later that morning, Raymond was supposed to have the information about the limousine service for my mother. As the clock reached 10, then 10:30am, and with the wedding starting at 3 p.m., my mom and I began to panic.

So what do you know, I ended up driving around the corner to see what was going on. As I came into the house, I was surprised to see he was actually still asleep. I slapped him lightly on the face and poured cold water on him to get up. He had a hangover from the bachelor party, the night before. I asked him about the money and the limousine, but he acted like he didn't know what I was talking about. We got into a big argument. I mean, we literally cussed each other out just hours before the wedding. I felt like there was no turning back now; after all the money my mother spent on this wedding, I was going through with this. One of the groomsmen had arrived at the door, so I left. I don't even remember what I said before I left. We didn't hug or kiss, say "I love you," none of that. I remember leaving with my heart bleeding, frustrated and deceived, and had shed so many unhappy tears. Larry, the groomsman, encouraged him to get ready for the big day and to think positive. I drove back over to my mother's house and told her the situation. She tried to stay calm just for my sake. Mom suggested I call Kelly, one of my bridesmaids, a family friend, and the aide that took care of my grandmother for nine years. I swallowed my pride, called, and asked her for $250, and she said yes. I drove over to Kelly's house to get the money. I felt so embarrassed, like I wish I could've just hidden from everybody, but I kept going. My mom paid the majority of the balance, and his grandmother, Mrs. Perry, paid about $200. We rented a stretch Lincoln Navigator. The cost was about $850. As the hour drew near, I started getting nervous. I asked God to forgive me for arguing with my soon-to-be husband before the wedding. I just concentrated on staying calm and thinking positive.

    I was beautiful, and started taking pictures before the wedding started. As I heard the music starting to play and as it got closer for me to walk down the aisle, I was so fucking nervous. My palms were sweaty, my heartbeat started to race faster and faster. I felt my head spinning, and I had to keep taking deep breaths and just concentrate on getting through this. I thought that since this moment was finally here, when we got married he would change, and things would be better; because after all, we're not shacking anymore, and it's better to be married than to burn. As I stood before the church doors, I was just ready to get it over with. I was honored and happy that my father was by my side. As I looked at my husband-to-be, I was thinking *yes, this is it*. This is what we had to do for it to get better, and knew he'd become a changed man. Raymond smiled a little bit, but showed no emotions as my dad gave me away, shedding some tears. Raymond looked as if he wanted to hurry up and get it over with too, but was trying to act like he wanted to be there. I can admit I felt the same way too. On one part of the vows, we both got tongued tied on the word ordinances. I looked over and my mother was crying, and everyone just looking, and I'm saying to myself, *what are these people thinking*? I could just imagine some of the things people were saying in their minds. We both sounded low as we repeated back and forth, and when it came time for us to kiss, it was a little kiss. I actually said to myself, *I wanted better than that,* and then I actually heard someone repeat those words out loud.

    After my Pastor announced us husband and wife and it was time for us to exit the church, I was so relieved. It's like we both could've run out the church. We greeted the guests as usual, and had to take pictures inside. It rained cats and dogs all day and night. We had apologized to each other for earlier that morning. We were all right from the time we got in the limo and to the reception. I felt like I was starting to go through the motions. I was playing a role that I was a happy bride and everything was okay, but it wasn't. Everyone seemed like they had a good time, but there was one person missing from the whole thing—my Aunt Charmaine. Sometime before the wedding she wrote me a note, warning me not to be disobedient, not to go along with this wedding. She said she loved me very much, but she wouldn't support it because it was not of God. She said if I went along with this wedding, I would be headed for a road to destruction.

That night after the reception, Raymond suggested that we have some company over to our house, watch some movies, and order something to eat. Some of the bridesmaids and groomsmen came over. I was so disappointed, but didn't show it. I thought, *Who in their right mind invites company over on their wedding night*? While everyone was downstairs, I went upstairs to take off my wedding dress. I thought he would follow me up. I actually had to call him upstairs and ask him to unzip me. I wanted to be alone with my husband. I was frustrated at everybody else for the simple fact they didn't go home, but it wasn't their fault. He practically begged them to hang out with us.

We didn't consummate or make love any that night. I cried as I took off my wedding dress. I thought to myself, *this is just the beginning to the road of my destruction.*

Within the next month and some odd weeks, I didn't feel right. I felt something was going on with my body. I was starting to have a foul odor and discharge when I went to the bathroom. One night when Raymond stayed out late past 3 or 3:30 in the morning, I was glad. I was led to call into work sick that morning. I had to work the day shift from 7 to 3 p.m., but I acted like I was going into work anyway. I was up my usual time, put my work clothes on, and left the house with my scrubs on. I don't remember if he came home that morning before I left or not.

I went downtown to kill some time then I was led to go to the emergency room so I could find out what was going on. After I was checked in, the Doctor gave me a pelvic exam and took some cultures. When she came back in the room, she asked me if I had been using protection. I told her no, and that I was married. She told me I had a Sexually Transmitted Disease (STD), chlamydia, and she would have to give me a shot, and then I would be okay. I had to lie on my stomach. The needle itself seemed like a foot long and she had to stick it in my butt cheek. She gave me some Tylenol for the soreness.

I felt like I didn't want to live. I felt like somebody took all my insides out and stomped all over them. We weren't even married two months. When I got back home, I got right into my pajamas and went straight to bed. It felt good to just lie down and rest my head. I was thinking what I would tell him when he came home. About an hour or so later, I heard these voices from a car outside, and one of them was Raymond's voice. The bedroom window was cracked. He was describing how he had some woman positioned, and how she looked. I felt like I was being buried alive. As a matter of fact, he was supposed to be at work. He was working at Big D's, a beauty supply store on West Main Street. I didn't hear anything else they talked about except for when he said goodbye to the other man he was talking with. I heard him walk in the house and take Sincere, our pit bull puppy, outside. I stayed in bed. I felt numb as ever.

Approximately twenty minutes later, I heard him come back in with Sincere. I knew he had company because he was talking to someone as he put the puppy away in the basement. I couldn't hear exactly what he was saying; I just know he was talking and nobody was talking back to him. I wondered who in the world he was talking to. I started to hear the person mumble back. It sounded like the person couldn't talk for some reason, and it was muffled. I continued to lie in the bed, like I was led to do.

Suddenly I heard him run up the stairs. Oh my goodness, he was butt-naked, nothing but socks on. The way the bed was positioned, facing the door, he should have seen me in the bed as soon as he entered the bedroom. I had the sheets and comforter over me, but still, he should have seen me. Not only that, my flannel brown and black sweater that I wear out just about every day was hanging on the door, in clear view. My work uniform was lying at the foot of the bed, and my work sneakers were by the door. He didn't see anything. I saw him come into the bedroom butt-naked, go into the dresser drawer, and get a condom or two. My goodness, I felt like my whole body was on fire. I started to shake, and I felt like I had a fireball inside my stomach as I heard the noises coming from downstairs. I could hear his deep voice like he was telling her to do something. I had no idea what I was going to do.

About three minutes later, I got out of the bed quietly, tiptoed to the stair case, and ran swiftly down the stairs. They jumped up quickly. They both looked as if they were going to die. He was standing in front of me with the condom on. She was half-naked on the couch. Oh my God, this was a deaf woman he was fucking. That would explain the mumbling and the conversing back and forth I found in his notebook. I punched him in the face without hesitation when he started to speak.

"I deserve that," Raymond said shamefully. The woman tried to sneak out, and I ran after her, but he grabbed me as he threw her purse to her. She yelled sorry as she ran out the door. I wondered what in the world did he see in her. She was fat and had a jerry curl, unattractive altogether. I scratched, screamed, punched, to get away from him, and I did. I tried and wanted to kill him. I took the lamp in the living room and threw it at him. He tried to talk, but I wasn't having it.

"Baby, I'm sorry." He ran into the kitchen. I grabbed a steak knife and threatened to use it on him. This answered my question as to why or how someone could commit murder. I was foaming at the mouth, and my adrenaline was at its highest peak.

*CRASH!*

The glass from the back door broke everywhere when my fist went through it. I felt no pain, except in my heart. My heart had a lot of pain. All I wanted to do was hurt him, make him feel what I was feeling.

I heard the next-door neighbors come outside. About five minutes later, the police arrived. Raymond explained to them the situation, and I just broke down. One officer asked me to come outside. The officer asked me if I was hurt, and did I need an ambulance? I told him no. Raymond came and stood beside me. The first word he tried to speak, I stopped him by giving him a hard-ass punch in the face. Yes, in front of the cops. The cop grabbed my fist and said, "Ma'am, I said no one is to be putting their hands on anybody. Mr. Wilson, would you like to press charges?"

"No, officer," Raymond replied.

"Okay, one of you guys needs to leave so you can calm down. Mr. Wilson, do you have somewhere you can go for a few hours?"

"Yes Officer, I'll leave."

Officer Frank walked me in the house. By the look on his face, the officer was saddened by the situation.

"How long have you been married?" Officer Frank asked.

"Barely two months," I cried.

"I'm sorry to hear that. Are you going to be okay?"

"Yes, Officer."

"Okay, I think you need to get some rest."

"Yes, thank you." As I shut the door, the feeling I had was unexplainable. I couldn't eat, and didn't dare call anybody. I just cried myself to sleep. All this happened a week or so before my birthday, August 23rd. Around this time, I went downtown to take the ASVAB, the army placement exam. I passed, got up and went to Buffalo, New York for a night or two for the physical. I had passed everything up until the eye exam. They sent me to three different eye doctors. My left eye was weak. When they gave me the eye exams, I was reading from the right eye instead of the left. The doctor with the say-so was the doctor that would pass me to the next step of the physical. He told me they would pay for me to have surgery done, or I could just resign. I decided to take advantage of the opportunity to resign. I returned back home to Rochester.

Raymond said he was praying I would return home, and that I didn't join the army. I left him a letter before I left while he was out somewhere, stating where I was going and what I was doing. Not long after that, we were getting evicted. We had no place to stay together. My mom and stepdad didn't want him at their house, nor his mother or grandparents. I stayed with my mom and Raymond said he was staying at his cousins or one of his homeboy's houses. At this point, it felt like we were just friends dating. We didn't see each other every day. Sometimes I would call for him on the cell phone or pager, and it would take him forever to call me back. I was starting to see less and less of him.

One night while at my mom's house, all of us were distracted by someone honking in the driveway. It was a white Honda Accord. We were all shocked. I was glad he got a car, but the question in my mind was, how did he get it? He took me with him that night. He drove us all the way to Syracuse, New York. He took a couple of bills from a stash, then went inside a convenience store. I opened the compartment between the driver and passenger seat, counted the stash. It was about $500.

"How'd you get this?" I asked him when he got back in the car.

"Never mind," Raymond said.

I just left it alone. We went to a motel with a Jacuzzi. While trying to make love to him in the Jacuzzi, I couldn't get into it. It felt like he wasn't making love to me. It was like he wanted me to be somebody else. As I looked at his arm between his shoulder and elbow, I spotted a hickey.

"What the hell is this?" I asked Raymond loudly.

"It ain't nothing. What are you talking about?"

I immediately got out of the water. He denied it was a hickey, but I knew better.

He was good about bringing me dinner at work when I asked him to. I was working 3-11 p.m. this one night, and he bought me Popeye's on my lunch break. Oh yeah, by the way, he admitted to me over dinner one night that he was selling drugs, and it was what he had to do. But that night he was supposed to pick me up at 11 p.m. It wasn't unusual for him to be thirty, forty-five minutes, or an hour late picking me up. It got to be 11:30, then 12:30 a.m. I kept calling and calling his cell phone, but I could tell he had it off because the voicemail kept coming on right away. It was about 1:00am when I left work. I felt like I could just die. I didn't want to call anybody for a ride, and even though I could have, I didn't. My mom had a car, and Uncle D, who was staying with Mom, still had his Jeep Cherokee. They were barely fifteen minutes away, where I worked at Hill Haven as per-diem on Empire Boulevard.

It was a straight shot, Clifford Avenue to Empire Boulevard, but it wasn't a good walk. I only had my brown and black flannel sweater, and it got as low as 25 degrees that night. Empire Boulevard had no sidewalks, there were hardly any street lights, with wooded areas. At the time, I didn't care what happened to me. I was too embarrassed to let my family know that my husband left me stranded and I didn't feel like hearing their opinions.

About 4 o'clock that morning, I got a phone call from Raymond. He sounded all serious, like he was in trouble. He asked me to ask my mother for her car to take him to the emergency room. He said that a taxi was dropping him off where I was, which was at my mom's house. My first thought was, *Why can't the taxi take us to the hospital*? I asked her and told him, but she wasn't trying to hear it. When he got there, I prayed that he was okay. When I got in the taxi, I could tell he was in a lot of pain.

"What in the world happened to you? Are you all right?"

"I'll be all right. I just paid this man $200 to drive me all the way from Canada. I'll tell you all about it later."

It took us about ten minutes to get to the hospital, not even. While Raymond was being seen by the triage nurse, he said he fell down some stairs, and that he was just in a lot of pain. When a room finally became available 15-20 minutes later, Raymond passed out. I could tell he'd been drinking a lot. I started to check him over myself. I knew he had gotten into some trouble. I saw someone's fingerprints on his arm, chest, and parts of his shoulder. Whoever this person was literally tried to hold him down for dear life. He had this big abrasion on nearly the whole left side of his back. I knew something much worse happened than him just falling down some stairs.

When the doctor finally came in to check him out, he couldn't get Raymond to wake up. He was so drunk it took us minutes to wake him.

When we finally did, he couldn't hold a conversation clearly. The doctor asked him what happened. He told him the same thing. I don't remember how he said he fell down the stairs, but the doctor gave him some solution to drink so he could do a CAT scan to check for any broken bones or internal bleeding. There were no broken bones or internal bleeding. It turned out that he had some swollenness in certain areas. Part of his shoulder was swollen. The doctor gave him a shoulder restraint and prescribed him some pain medication. His mother had let him stay with her a couple of days, and he got some family support when they found out he had been hurt.

Raymond finally told me the real deal. He and some friends rented a limo and went over to Niagara Falls, Canada. He said he got into an argument with a man in Burger King, and security tried to hold him down, but he got away. He ran through alleys and tried to jump from one roof to another, but he missed and fell in a ditch, and he couldn't get out. He yelled out to one of his friends, who heard him and helped him out of the ditch. That's when he found a taxi and got away. He bragged and bragged about the fact that he was able to get away. I was glad that he didn't get caught and that he was okay.

I knew that he'd been sleeping with other people. I could just feel it. Then there were the things he'd say to me when we did have sex, like that I wasn't doing it right, or demanding me to watch porno flicks so I could do it like they did in the movie. One night he took me out to a club, and I had some drinks. When we left I dozed off in the car. He thought I passed out. He drove to the house of one of his ex-girlfriends, Cathy, while I was still in the car. After he pulled into the driveway, he got out hesitantly, and went into the house. Before we left, they exchanged some words, and she said, "She's knocked out cold."

"She's drunk," Raymond replied.

I was awake the whole entire time.

"I thought you was asleep," he said as he drove away.

"Every shut eye ain't closed," I told him.

"So why did you look like you were sleeping?"

He looked pissed off and like he wanted to hit the window. I didn't say a word. He said that she was keeping the puppy for him, because he didn't have anywhere else to take it. After he told me that, I had my doubts that he'd been messing around with her.

On Christmas day that year, I hadn't seen him the whole day, not until the early evening. He came by my mother's house, where I was still staying at the time. He'd bought me a gold chain with a heart, elephant bracelet and a ring. He also gave me long stem roses made of glass. I thought it was weird, because he didn't give me a vase to put them in, nor did we have our own place. What seemed even weirder, he gave me a burgundy leather coat that was three times my size. He said he bought it that big so I could have it a long time, and plus, when I got pregnant I'd still be able to wear it. Something did not sit right with me about that, because he had bought me a coat before and he knew my correct size.

I don't remember getting him anything. If I did, it wasn't anything as expensive as the two $500 Avirex leather coats he'd gotten. His grandmother bought him one when she went to New York City, and he bragged and bragged about it. He was already wearing the Avirex his grandmother bought him, and to remind you, we were still at my mother's house. What hurt me so bad, and embarrassed me, was that he bragged about a gift his friend Tammy bought for him. The same friend he'd lied and said was his cousin. My brothers, sister, mother, and uncle knew she had to be more than just a friend, as they saw it was a leather Avirex as he pulled it out of the box. My heart bled so heavy. I wanted to cry as he said, "I have friends like that."

*Perpetuality*

I wanted to hide under a rock. Everyone looked as if they were surprised I would accept that from him. I tried as hard as I could to control my expressions and body language.

"You wouldn't want any guy friends buying anything for her," my mother said, trying to keep her cool.

"She don't have any guy friends," Raymond replied.

We went to her house after he embarrassed me at my mother's. "Why'd you buy it so big?" his grandmother asked.

"I bought it big so when she gets pregnant, she'll have enough room." Mrs. Perry laughed.

"Look at what Tammy bought me," Raymond said.

"What is another woman doing buying you a gift?"

"Grandma, she's just a good friend."

"Umm-hmm.

I couldn't believe what I was hearing.

Cathy, the ex-girlfriend who was keeping the puppy for Raymond, had an uncle who worked at the same security company as my stepdad Melvin and my Uncle D, who was still staying with my mother also. Cathy's uncle was gossiping about the conversations he overheard Cathy having with her aunt about a guy named Golden, not knowing that Golden is Raymond's nickname. Neither did he know he was repeating everything he heard to my family. Cathy was saying how good it felt when he ate her out, and how he had her in different positions, and she loved when he gave it to her doggy style. Cathy's aunt had told her how she heard them getting it on in the other room, and she heard her saying his name. I overheard my uncle and stepdad talking to my mother. They didn't know I was there listening. I literally just broke down, and felt so alone. I felt like I deserved everything that was happening.

Around this time, Raymond found us a place to stay on Priscilla Street. It was a house for rent, just around the corner from my mother and also not far from where his grandparents lived. One evening, Raymond and I went to visit my mother Vanessa. While Raymond went upstairs to play PlayStation with my brothers Adam and Andre, I checked his leather coat pockets, because I just knew he was being unfaithful. I found two 5x7 pictures of an unknown female. She was very attractive. I turned a picture over, and on the back it said, "To Golden, my man, stay sweet, love Hannah." He had left his pager in the coat as well. It was a pager that received text messages. I checked the messages, and he had a few from Cathy about taking her to an auto parts store, asking him to stop by, what time, and what time to meet her. After that I saw an *I love you* message, and what time to be by her place to take her to the mall. That message was from Hannah. He was also receiving messages from Tammy to please call her. I didn't approach him about this yet. I didn't want to hear him lie and give me excuses.

One night, I went bowling with my sister Lauren and some of her friends from work. I decided to call Hannah's number from a pay phone to see if he would answer, since I knew it by heart from his pager. I hung up as soon as I recognized his voice.

At our new house we were renting, nothing had changed. It grew worse and worse. Some nights when he said he was going out with the fellas, or going out to hustle, I had him drop me off at my mother's house until he was done. It would be embarrassing at times because he wouldn't pick me back up until six or seven o'clock in the morning, and I didn't have a key to get in my own house even if my family offered to take me home. When I did stay home, he didn't come back home until eleven o'clock the next day or afternoon. Those were the nights I called every hospital and jail in the city, after calling some of

## Perpetuality

his family to find out if they saw him. One day as we lay together, I noticed he had scratches on his chest and on his back. I knew I didn't do it, because I had on acrylic nails, and they don't scratch unless they're broken. When I asked him about it, he said one of his boys did it while they were wrestling.

"Why would I come home with scratches on me?" Raymond asked me.

I said nothing else. I would still check his pager from time to time by calling the toll-free number and asking the operator the messages and who they were from. I knew his passcode, because one day I saw him key it in on his cell phone while he didn't know I was looking. He had phone numbers galore on pieces of paper from different females. I would find condoms and receipts from hotels.

One Sunday morning after getting off a night shift, I decided to just catch the bus home, since he wasn't there to pick me up. I wanted to go to church, and I had to sing in the choir. When I got off the bus and got closer to the house, I had a funny feeling, because his car was there. My first thought was he had another hangover, and overslept. As I walked upstairs it was quiet. I walked into our bedroom, and I could've passed out. I stood there, wishing it was a dream. I said to myself, "Oh no, this can't be real." I went back downstairs to the kitchen, and said "Lord help me, Holy Ghost, help me." I couldn't scream. I couldn't cry. Raymond was in the bed naked with a fat, dark-skinned female, and not only that, there was a young man lying in a pivot position at the foot of the bed. There were used condoms on the floor, and an empty E&J bottle. No one heard me walk in the room, and they didn't hear me the first time, until I called his name.

"Raymond. Raymond!" He still didn't hear me. The young man at the foot of the bed and the fat woman that was lying next to him both woke up. The young man pushed and pulled at Raymond until he woke up. The lady didn't know what to say. She just repeated what the young man had said. Raymond, on the other hand, swore on his grandmother's grave, his cousin's grave, that he didn't do anything. The young man said what happened was that he and the lady did have sex, but Raymond was knocked out cold, and he didn't do anything. He should've kept his mouth shut, because he either didn't know or had forgotten there was an extra bedroom right next to the master bedroom. The question in my mind was, why would you come and have sex on the bed when he's already naked in the bed, unless all three of them were having a ménage à trois, which I knew had happened. In the midst of them being caught and trying to get dressed at the same time, I saw them trying to pick up the used condoms on the sneak tip. The Holy Ghost really dealt with me then, because I said, "I ain't mad at ya. Y'all need Jesus. I forgive you all."

Raymond was going to give them a ride home. I asked him to bring me some stockings back for church. He insisted that I go with them. I said no. Then he demanded me to. I felt weird and awkward getting in the car with everybody. He drove me to the store first. I wish I had a recorder to hide in the car, because I knew they were all talking and planning while I was inside. I don't remember where he dropped off the young man. The woman got dropped off at a house or apartment. When she got to the door, he pulled off. I don't believe she stayed there.

"Are you okay, Boo?"

"I'm fine."

We both went to church that morning like a happy married couple as if nothing happened, and I knew the only reason he went was he thought it would make me feel better.

A few months later, I received a phone call late at night. It was Raymond, calling from jail. He told me to come downtown to the jail and see him because I didn't have to schedule the first visit, which was Saturday, because he didn't have long to talk and he only had one phone call, which was only five minutes. The next day I went to go visit him. He said he had got caught with a gun in the car.

"How did they catch you?" I asked.

"The cop said I had run a stop sign. I told him I was looking both ways."

Raymond had two other men with him at the time. One of them was my cousin David. I believe he said one of them tried to run, and something didn't sound right with the cop. They were put in different police cars, when more cops showed up. The car was searched, and a gun was found in between the passenger and driver's seat. Raymond's bail was set for $2,500. Everyone from his Grandmother, my mother, and myself paid, pawning the jewelry he bought for me, and my wedding ring he told me to pawn. On top of that, he had arranged for me to sell the rims off his Honda Accord, for $900, to one of his friends. It took about six weeks to come up with the bail money. I had $1900, and he told me when he called to meet his brother downtown at the jail, because he would have the rest of the money. I had my mother drive me. When I got to the desk to bail Raymond out, I saw his brother along with Cathy and Hannah.

"Well, I might as well introduce myself. I'm Hannah, and you must be Allana?"

"Yes, I am."

"And I'm Cathy."

After we said hello to each other, we realized all three of us were getting played, and his brother knew the same.

"I'm not in it, I just did what he told me to."

His brother Lucas had been honest about the fact that Cathy was going to come with him. She didn't want to just give him $500. I don't know if he knew about Hannah showing up or not. There was no need for me to get mad at either of these women. For one, he wasn't worth it, and I had to blame myself for letting him treat me the way he did. True indeed, we all were getting played. All three of us went down to the part of the jail where he would be released. His brother Lucas left and didn't want to stay. While we were waiting on him, they told me everything, starting with Hannah.

I found out she was Jamaican by her accent, and that he had been having unprotected sex with her on top of saying that he wanted her to have his baby, and even mentioned wedding plans to her. She said she found my ID in his green wallet, and she asked him who I was, and he said that we were cousins. She said she saw his wedding ring in the compartment between the passenger and driver's seat, but that he still denied he was married. I knew if she didn't know he was married in the beginning, she knew somewhere down the line. Cathy said that she had given him the money to buy his Honda Accord, his wedding ring, and gave him money to start hustling. She even told me that the elephant bracelet and the burgundy leather coat, along with the glass stem roses, he had bought for her. That's why it seemed weird to me at the time. Raymond got mad and took it from her when they had an argument. They both admitted to me that he took them both to Cor Joes, a strip joint, to have a ménage à trois with one of the strippers, on separate occasions. They said they chose not to do it, but I didn't believe them. Cathy and Hannah both could describe our house and everything in it. Everything, all the way down to our bedroom sheets. Cathy said she had gotten pregnant, but she had a miscarriage. I found out that he had been staying with Tammy at times also. They both knew about Tammy. Raymond used her apartment to perform his sexual acts when she was at work. Cathy said she couldn't believe he had gotten married. She wasn't the first person I had heard say that.

"I could've gotten married to him if I wanted to, when we were together, but I didn't," Cathy stated. They had dated about five or six years prior.

"That's your husband," Hannah said.

"If I were you, I would get a divorce," Cathy replied.

As he walked down the hall, I could tell by Raymond's face he didn't know whether to run or keep walking. He looked at me with a sorry-ass look on his face as they both cussed him out.

"And you got the nerve to be carrying the Bible," Cathy said with disgust.

"Thank you, but I'll give you both your money back."

I walked away without saying anything. I shoved him as he grabbed me.

"You don't have anything to say?"

"Fuck you. I'll be packing my stuff, and by the way, I know you don't think you're riding in my mother's car." If I had my own car and drove myself, I would have taken him. I know how foolish I was.

"How am I supposed to get home? I just got out of jail."

"Figure it out."

I walked away and all three of us ended up talking with my mother, who had stayed in the car the whole time. They basically were repeating some of the things they told me. Hannah said that he was getting attached to her three-year-old child and everything. She was very hurt. She shed a couple of tears. She was angry at herself for believing him.

My mother encouraged us all. She said we didn't need to put up with that. We all agreed how he looked, as he stood at the door, figuring out how he was going to get home. My mother drove me to my and Raymond's house to get my stuff. It wasn't too much longer, a day or two, that I was back with him.

After him being released from jail, I knew he continued to keep in touch with both women. The money that they put up for him to get out of jail was their reason to stay in touch.

Later on in the summer, I went on a cruise with my mother Vanessa, my sister Lauren, and my brothers Adam and Andre, and my Aunt Charmaine. We went to the Bahamas. I was in no shape to pay for the cruise, except I helped pay for the plane ticket. I never kept money or was ever able to get anything for myself. Raymond didn't want me to go on the cruise, but I went anyway. I knew I needed to get away. If I hadn't gone, I probably would have had an emotional breakdown. I was already depressed and distressed.

As he drove me to the airport, I remember him banging on the dashboard, calling me a "stupid-ass bitch." I ignored him. What I remember so very well was the hateful, demonic, mean look in his eyes as he said he hoped that the plane I got on would crash. I could've just broken down, but I kept it together for the sake of my mother and stepdad, and everybody else we would meet at the airport.

A couple of days later, I couldn't believe it—I heard a news broadcast that the R&B singer Aaliyah had been killed because her plane crashed not too far from where we were vacationing. I said *Thank you, Lord. It could've been me.*

I called Raymond a couple of times when I wasn't on the boat. It was less expensive. All I got was his voicemail. I didn't worry about it. I set my mind on just having a ball. I told every guy that approached me that I was married. At first I did take my ring off, but I put it back on. Two wrongs don't make a right. It was so refreshing to be on the sandy white beaches and in the clear blue water. Even just looking at the ocean while I was on the boat was very restoring to me. It was like my soul and everything in me was being replenished.

*Perpetuality*

We'd just started staying with my mother before I left for the cruise. We had a garage sale, and sold all our furniture, down to the computer for $3500. His so-called plan was to move us to Georgia. I still don't know where the money went. One morning, I woke up and decided to see what was on the tape recorder I had found in the compartment between the driver's and passenger seat. He was fast asleep, as he always was when he would drink. As I listened to the tape, he was having sex talk with Hannah. He was asking her to tell him how she feels when he makes love to her. I heard them even talk about marriage, and around the time they should plan. Everything about sexual positions, from doggy style, oral, and anal sex, was on the tape. I don't remember who was at home at the time, but I couldn't wait to return to the attic where we slept. He was already awake.

"What the hell is this?" I yelled.

"What the hell are you talking about?" he replied, looking at the recorder in my hand.

"Oh, now you got goddamn amnesia now? You don't remember what's on the tape, with you and Hannah?"

"I'm not even with Hannah anymore. If you want you can call and ask her. That's in the past. So why are you bringing the past up?"

Get the fuck out, Raymond," I screamed as I threw the recorder at him.

"You can't tell me to get out. This is not your house," he said with a smirk on his face.

"I can't stand your ass. You need to quit acting phony. You don't even want to stay here. I want you to leave."

"Whatever, you stupid ass bitch. You need to shut the fuck up." He stepped to me and balled up his fist, as if he was going to punch me in the face.

I kept my composure the best I could, because this was my mother's and step-dad's house. Not too long after that, about a few days or so, he finally left, after one night he saw that I didn't want to be bothered with him. When I was studying, he acted like he was trying to help me, and telling me how I should do my homework. I didn't want his help, and my actions showed it very much. He got pissed off and said, "That's why I've been cheating." He said he was going to start cheating again. He drove away that night and didn't come back. He didn't care what my mother or stepdad thought about it.

The next time I clearly remember seeing him was on 9/11. Yes, when the twin towers were hit, which was just days after the night he left. I was in my Psychology 101 class at the time, and we got an announcement that we needed to vacate the building. It took about two hours to get home, when it usually only took about 15 minutes. I carpooled with two other students that day. During this tragedy, I prayed that Raymond was okay. When I finally got to my mother's house, he called and came by to pick me up. It did make me feel good that he called to see if I was okay. Even though it happened four hours away, it still had an impact. But instead of acting like husband and wife, I felt like I was just dating or just a plaything to Raymond.

## Chapter Four

I didn't tell Raymond that I had gone to see about getting a new car. It had been weeks prior, when my Aunt Charmaine took me to Webster Chrysler Jeep to see if I would qualify for a new vehicle, a red Plymouth Neon 2001. I ended up having a black salesman by the name of Bobby Blake. He asked me what I wanted, and I told him straight off the bat, "A red Plymouth Neon." He told me if I put $100 down, he could start processing my application. I told him I didn't have it, but that maybe I could get it from my aunt when she got back from Wal-Mart, across the street. He offered to pay $10 out of his own pocket to start the process. I accepted.

"Lana, telephone."

"Hello?"

"Hi, Allana, this is Bobby Blake. How are you doing today?"

"Fine, how are you?"

"Listen, I was calling to see if you had a trade-in."

I thought for a minute. "Well, I had a Pontiac Sunbird, but me and my dad towed it to the Vanderstyne Ford dealership a while ago, out in Greece, when I thought I was going to get a car out there, but it didn't work out."

"Do you have someone who can take you out there?"

"No, I won't be able to get out there right now."

"Okay, let me see what I can do. I'll call you back, okay?"

"Okay."

I picked up the phone when it rang this time. It was Bobby Blake.

"Hello?"

"Hi, yes, is this Allana?"

"Yes it is," I said in a soft voice.

He chuckled. "I can give you a ride out to the dealership, where you said your car is. Can you be ready in about fifteen minutes?"

"Yes, I sure will. Thank you very much." I tried not to sound as excited as I was. I thought, *Oh my goodness, this is such a blessing.* I couldn't believe how this man I hardly knew wanted to really help me out. A thought did come to my mind that I should call Raymond, because I was riding with another man without his permission, but I thought about it again, and said, "I don't think so." This was the next day after he decided to get up and leave, after I ignored and acted like I didn't want to be bothered with him. I hadn't seen or heard from him all night and day. It was late afternoon when Bobby showed up to take me to the Vanderstyne Ford Dealership to see if my old car was still there.

Raymond had come out to Webster Chrysler one time with me so I could show him what car I wanted, and he had met Bobby as well. He was nonchalant about it.

I was good and ready when Bobby came to the door. *What a gentleman*, I thought as we walked to the car.

"Thank you very much. She really needs a car," my mom said, standing in the doorway, watching us walk to the car.

"I'm going to make sure of that," Bobby replied.

"Where's what's-his-name, Raymond, your husband? He didn't want to come?"

I just shrugged my shoulders. "I haven't seen him."

Bobby looked at me with a confused look on his face. "Okay." While on our way to the car dealership, we had casual conversation. I told him I was working as a Nursing Assistant, and was going to school to become a nurse. Most of the time I was quiet, staring out the window. I was embarrassed, for one, that another man was taking me to handle business Raymond should have been handling. That was obvious, and I was so tired and depressed inside.

*Perpetuality*

"Hey, you're in a different world over there. What are you thinking? What's on your mind? Are you okay?"

"I'm okay. Thank you."

I found it amazing that he really wanted to know what I was thinking about. I felt like killing myself, taking a bunch of pills, and calling it quits.

"I was just thinking about some things I'm going through with Raymond. I'm tired, so tired." I felt like breaking down. My eyes got watery, but I held it in the best I knew how.

Bobby could tell I was in a bad situation and that I wasn't happy. It really showed. I felt him come into my world a little bit, when he asked me my thoughts. When we arrived at the dealership, he went inside to ask a few salesmen about my old car still being there. He came back outside, with no luck. We looked all over from the front to the back of the car lot, but there was no Pontiac Sunbird. So, we left and had to go with another plan. It had been six, seven months, maybe almost a year, since I had left the white Pontiac Sunbird there after the transmission blew out on me at two in the morning while I was exiting a pitch black highway, going to Windsor Gardens, the apartment we had just moved into on Manitou Road. Raymond and I had both worked as janitors at night at Kodak, through Kelly's Temp Services, after not staying that long at JC Penney in Greece Ridge Mall. Thank God I had a cell phone at the time. Raymond came to the rescue in his Green Plymouth Breeze.

"Are you hungry? Would you like something to eat?" Bobby asked.

"Sure."

"Where do you want to go?" he asked, leaving the decision totally up to me.

"Burger King or McDonald's is fine."

He grinned at me and said, "Where do you really want to go?" I looked around and saw Olive Garden, one of my favorite restaurants.

"Olive Garden would be nice," I said shyly. I was feeling a vibe with this man, and didn't really know where it was going, but I was definitely attracted to him. I was a little nervous, but became more comfortable when we talked and got to know one another. He asked me my age, and I asked his. I was 24 at the time, and he was 35.

"Do you have kids?" Bobby asked.

"No, I don't. Thank God. Do you have kids?" I returned the question.

"I have an eight-year-old and sixteen-year-old, both girls. I love them very much and am so very proud of them."

"Awww. That's sweet," I said, adoring the fact that he loved his kids.

About two days later, he called me at about 9:30 a.m. "Hey, Allana. How are you?"

"Fine. How are you?" I said, feeling nervous at the same time, wondering what plan he came up with so I could drive off the lot.

"Okay, all I need you to do is come up with $120 down on the car, and you can drive off today. Do you think you can do that?"

"Yes," I said hesitantly, not knowing where I was going to get the money.

"Can I call you back in ten minutes?"

"Okay, ten minutes."

"Mommy," I called to her in an excited voice.

"What?"

"Mommy, do you have $120? Bobby said I can drive off the lot today, if I put it down on the car."

"What?" she said with a smile on her face. "When am I going to get it back?" she said jokingly. "Will they take a check?"

"I don't know. They should. Let me call him back." I dialed Bobby's number again. "Yes, hi. Could you transfer me to Bobby Blake please?"

"Sure. One moment."

"This is Bobby, how may I help you?"

"Hey Bobby, it's Allana."

"Hey."

"Would it be okay if my mom wrote a check?"

"Yes, that's fine. The only thing I'll need is her ID, and I need you to be ready in about thirty minutes. Is that all right with you?"

"Yes. I don't have to be to school until 12 p.m."

"The only reason I say that is because I have to get this done today."

"Okay. Thank you, Bobby."

"You're welcome, and I'll see you soon."

I felt like shouting through the whole house. I was going to be driving a new Plymouth Neon off the showroom, and it was red, my favorite color. My mother was happy for me. I thanked, hugged, and kissed her as she handed me the check and her license. Bobby didn't have to come to the door. I met him halfway. I brought my school books along with me.

"It's good to see you smiling," Bobby said when we got in the car.

"It feels so good to finally get my own car."

"So, what time did you say you had to be to school?"

"12 p.m."

"Okay, well I can drop you off and pick you back up, because we have to see where you're going to get your car insurance. State Farm is pretty good."

"Oh yes. I've had State Farm before. I'm fine with that."

When we got to the dealership, I had to sign a bunch of paperwork. I took a good look at the car again. Bobby told me that the Plymouth Neon on the floor inside the dealership was the only Neon they had in red. The other colors they had, I didn't care for. To my surprise, the red Neon, brand spanking new, never driven, was a stick shift. I felt like I was learning another language. All this about financing and getting a car loan was new to me. I just wanted to drive. My car note was $340 a month. Bobby was running around like a chicken with his head cut off, trying to get my paperwork done along with other things he had to do. He stopped and realized it was time for me to get to school.

"Man, you are busy," I told him when he came back to the table. "Take it easy."

He smiled.

When he picked me up from school, we headed straight to State Farm, not too far from the dealership. He had the appointment already set up. I felt a sense of security from a man who wasn't my father for the first time. When we went inside State Farm and talked to Mark, the insurance agent, the process took about twenty-five minutes. We headed back to Webster Chrysler Jeep, where my wheels were waiting for take-off. I was so excited, but at the same time I didn't want the process to end, still wanting to stay in touch with Bobby.

As I waited for my car to be taken outside from the showroom, Bobby said, "I know you can do it."

He was encouraging me that I knew how to drive stick shift. Judy, another salesperson said, "We can take you out and give you some lessons to get you comfortable, if you'd like."

"Thank you."

Bobby handed me the keys, then wrapped both his arms around me with a big hug and a kiss on the cheek to match. "You take care of yourself. If you need anything or have any questions, please don't be afraid to call."

"Thank you Bobby, for everything," I said as I walked away. I felt like I was floating on air. I screamed, "Thank you Jesus," when I got into my brand-new car.

About a day or two later, I purchased Bobby and Judy thank you cards. I wrote, "You are heaven sent," inside his card. They both weren't there, so I left each card on both their desks, and hoped I'd hear from Bobby soon.

"Hello?" It was Bobby.

"Hey, how are you doing?"

"Fine, and how are you?" I replied happily. I felt like I was melting, because I wanted to hear his voice.

"Um. I'm trying to think how I should say this."

I was just quiet. I didn't know what was going to come out of his mouth. My stomach was nervous.

"I've been thinking about you really hard. I think about you when I wake up and when I go to sleep. I'm thinking that you feel something between us."

"Yes."

I was surprised at what I was hearing.

"You're a smart and intelligent woman. You've got a lot going for yourself. I've never had feelings for a woman like this before. I had to let you know that I adore you, and thanks for the card. It really meant a lot to me."

"You're welcome."

He called me just about every day for about almost two months, from work, after work, even driving home, he'd call and talk to me through his Bluetooth. This man had me really thinking to move forward with my divorce, seriously, because Raymond had told me on various occasions that I wasn't shit and no other man would want me. I hadn't slept with this man and he treated me like a queen. He talked to me with respect, like I was a powerful woman. He made my mind feel so much better, emotionally he made me feel better, and I was starting to get really attached. We started spending time together.

On one particular date, he took me to a wine tasting out in the country, Wayne County. We ended up sleeping together for the first time. I was starting to feel guilty. I knew I couldn't play both sides of the fence.

One afternoon, he called me and asked me to meet him at Applebee's, about ten or fifteen minutes from me, and down the street from his job. Bobby said he would really like to talk and to see me. I borrowed one of my sister's outfits, that would give accent to my figure. I wore black fitted leather pants, with a turtle neck, and a black leather blazer. I took a deep breath before I went inside the restaurant.

"Hello Bobby."

He stood up and gave me a hug. He smelled so damn good. "Thanks for coming. Would you like something to eat?"

"No, thank you. A Sprite will be fine."

"Are you sure?"

"Yes, thank you." I knew I was lying through my teeth, knowing I wanted something to eat, but I played it off anyway.

"You look very beautiful."

"Thank you," I said in a shy tone, giggling.

"Allana, you make me feel good when I'm with you. I'm so comfortable. You're everything a man could ever ask for in a woman. I wasn't looking for it. You just, like, came out of nowhere and fell in my lap. I want to give you the world, if you let me. You don't deserve what you're going through."

*Perpetuality*

"Bobby, I really do thank you, but I'm still married, and I do want to try to work it out with Raymond. He's going to get help for his alcohol problem, and we're going to seek some counseling. I still love him."

"I can understand that, because he was your first love. He's a lucky man, but he doesn't deserve you. He takes you for granted, and I hate to see that."

I nodded my head, because everything he was saying was indeed true.

"Well, I wish you all the best, I really do."

"Thank you."

Bobby walked me to my car, gave me a hug, and put something in my hand. "You take care of yourself."

When I got in my car, I unfolded $40. I remembered that he asked me over the phone one day, how much it was to get my hair done, and I told him, not thinking for one moment, that he would give me the money. I called him later that evening and told him thank you. He told me I was very welcome, and that what he did was just the tip of the iceberg. I thought to myself, *What the hell am I doing?* I began to think I was selling myself short by staying with Raymond. Our marriage wasn't stable at all. So many times, countless times, I had separated from him.

Raymond had started calling me. One night he came to church, and I drove him and I to Charlotte Beach to talk. I told him about Bobby and me, and how we ended up sleeping together. Raymond took a deep swallow, and a deep breath. He asked if we used protection, and I said no. I was being honest, even though it was a bad decision. Raymond and I had been separated for about seven months at this time. He was telling me how God was changing him to be a better man, and how he wanted to provide for his family, but how hard it was because he had a felony.

"I love our marriage, and God put me to be the head of this marriage, but you have to trust me. I know it's hard, but you have to. I want us to start being honest with each other. I want to be able to tell you everything, and you tell me everything."

It was all the lovey-dubby stuff I wanted to keep hearing, because I simply didn't want to get a divorce. I wanted to stay married and live happily ever after.

"So, have you slept with anybody since we've been separated?" I asked him as he looked hesitant. "You might as well tell me. I know that you have."

"Yes, her name is Theresa, and she is a doctor. We have slept together more than a few times."

"How did you meet her?" I was feeling jealous he had to bring up the fact that she was a doctor.

"Me and Isaac was at the gas station on Portland and Clifford Ave. Isaac was like, 'Damn who is that?' She was driving a new white Escalade. I said 'Damn, she is drop dead gorgeous.' She was light-skinned, long pretty hair, and she had on jogging pants that showed her figure. She had a nice shape."

I looked at Raymond like he was crazy.

"Boo, it's not like that. I'm just being honest. I made a bet with Isaac that she would give me some play, and she did after I introduced myself like a gentleman, and I asked to pump her gas. I asked for her number, and she gave it to me. We started going out to dinner, and one thing led to another."

"Did you use protection?" I asked.

"No."

"So how the fuck are you going to get mad at me?"

*Perpetuality*

"Because you hardly know Bobby."

"And you know her so very well, right?"

He didn't have anything to say except, "All right, I don't want to argue. I want to start over the right way. I couldn't stay with Theresa because I was still in love with you."

What do you know, I was back with him for the, wait a damn minute, I don't know how many times. I couldn't tell you. I had already lost count.

\* \* \*

I was late getting back to the women's shelter. I had been staying at the Y for almost a month. Now that I knew I was back with Raymond, I didn't care about breaking any rules. The way I ended up at the Y was, one night Raymond got drunk. As we were leaving his grandparents' house, he asked me for the keys, and I told him, "You're not driving my car. You've been drinking." Raymond got mad, ran up to me with a threatening look on his face, and pushed me as I fell back. I gave a blood-curdling scream, like I was about to get killed. Mr. and Mrs. Perry ran outside. His grandmother tried to pull his hands off from around my neck as he choked me. After he pushed his grandmother, his grandfather got a hold of Raymond. He was literally fighting his grandfather.

"You don't be putting your hands on your grandmother, and that's your wife. What is wrong with you?" Mr. Perry yelled.

I got into the car as quickly as I could while Mr. Perry had a hold of him. I immediately locked my car doors. When I put the red Neon in reverse, Raymond was standing in back of the car, staring at me like he was Satan himself. He wouldn't budge. Mrs. Perry called the police. When the officer arrived, he asked if I was okay, and whose car it was.

After I proved to the officer that the car was in my name, I was free to go.

I was hysterical. I thought about driving off the road to kill myself. I decided to go to my Aunt Charmaine's house, after 1:00 in the morning. She opened her door and let me stay a couple of days, gave me a few therapy sessions until I checked into the Y, the women's shelter downtown.

Naïve and silly me. I let Raymond take my new car after he dropped me off at the Y, and said he'd be around the corner at his cousin Gary's house, who lived in the high-rise downtown on St. Paul Street across from World Wide News.

Again, I had disturbing peace in the pit of my stomach. I compromised and ignored it. After a day or so, he was late picking me up to take me to school. One Sunday morning, I went into the kitchen of the Y, the women's shelter, to look out the window to see if I could see my car parked at the Pinnacle Church of God in Christ. I was able to see the church and the parking lot from the shelter's kitchen. I could've walked to church, but I didn't want to be embarrassed with everyone asking me where my brand-new car was. I decided not to go to church that morning. I was so fucking pissed off. He never showed up with my car to take me to church, and knew I had to sing in the choir. I was absolutely disgusted. I saw him show up at the end of the service, then leave. When I asked him about it, he said he had gone to church and thought I was already there, but realized I wasn't when he saw my mother and sister, another dumbass story he made up that didn't make sense.

The shelter helped me get an apartment in Webster, but I wasn't due to move in for almost three weeks. Raymond was staying with his cousins, and I'm sure with other woman from time to time. Social Services put us up in a hotel together until we moved into the

*Perpetuality*

apartment. This was not your average comfortable or everyday hotel to stay in. The Cadillac Hotel was like a run-down, fucked-up boardinghouse for the homeless, infested with drug addicts, prostitutes, bed bugs, mice, and rats. So many mice, that I heard them crawling under the door at night, and under our bed where we slept. I reached over to turn on the lamp, and there were two climbing up the electric cord by the side of the bed. Oh my God, was I frantic. I put cardboard at the door thinking it would stop the mice from entering the room, but they just ate their way through it.

One morning I woke up, and it was a school day for me. Raymond had stayed out all night, and I didn't even receive a phone call. I was so sick with myself. I had to call Aunt Charmaine to come pick me up to take me to school.

We went ahead and moved into the apartment December 1st, out in Webster. Raymond and I hooked up the apartment really nice. After putting up wallpaper border, carpet, black leather couches, and other odds and ends, we made the apartment look like a penthouse, but none of that makes a home. This was our Christmas gift to each other, or to myself, I should say.

I worked like a Hebrew slave at the nursing home. Since I was working doubles back to back, nobody really ever saw me. I don't remember Raymond ever buying too much of anything for Christmas or birthdays. I can't think of one year we were settled to cook a Thanksgiving Turkey together. A home, that's something I never got from Raymond.

My grandmother passed right after the New Year came in. I was working the evening shift when my mom called me about 4 o'clock in the afternoon.

"Lana, she's gone."

I was—I can't explain it. I remember hanging up the phone. After I told my mom I was on my way, I called my Uncle D just in case Raymond didn't show up. They showed up at the same time. Rochester was starting to have lake effect snow that evening. Raymond asked me if I was okay, but I didn't feel support from him. I didn't believe it was genuine, just that he felt obligated. When Raymond and I pulled into my mother's driveway, I rushed right into the house.

I don't remember who I saw when I walked in the house. When I walked into the sunroom where my grandma's deathbed was, I laid my head on her chest, held her hand, and just cried and cried. I looked at her, and I was proud of her. I rubbed her braided hair. I knew someone from the other side had been laughing with her. She looked like she'd been laughing and talking with somebody from the look on her face.

My grandmother Annie Pearl Jackson was a trooper. I remember when she'd put me in the bathtub with her when I was a little girl. I remember her teaching me how to brush my teeth. She taught me how to say my prayers at night, and bless my food before I ate. One of my fondest memories is when she told me to open the bedroom screen window, and break off a switch for myself. I miss her wet kisses on my cheek.

On that same evening my grandmother passed, I thought I was going to be right behind her. Raymond was driving us home, and he had been drinking. We didn't have car insurance, and Raymond's license was suspended after too many speeding tickets. He got scared when he saw a Sheriff, and turned down a street off of Empire Boulevard. The roads had gotten very icy that night. This street he turned down led to a park. The road we were on started to curve. We crashed into the guardrail. I screamed as both my legs hit my chest, my head hit the dashboard, and then the headrest. We asked each other if

## Perpetuality

we were okay, but he was still paranoid about running into a cop. As Raymond started again, we ran into a dead end, nowhere to go. There was a lake, and a Sheriff already parked.

Raymond played it cool and got out the car to see what was damaged. He motioned for me to get out the car. The Neon was fucked up, a wreck, in the front. I was surprised we still had a headlight working, or that the car was still drivable. The Sheriff drove over to where we were, then two more Sheriff cars showed up. I wanted to run. As I prayed quietly to myself, the Sheriff asked what happened. I just knew we were going to jail after I knew he had already checked the license plates, but he said nothing about the car insurance being canceled. I let Raymond do all the talking. Raymond told the Sheriffs we simply lost control on the ice, and we had to change the flat tire. The other two Sheriffs left, and one stayed behind as Raymond changed the front tire. It was bitter cold out there. I thanked God over and over, for I knew my family couldn't handle another tragedy on top of my grandmother passing in the same night. When we finally arrived at the apartment, I despised him, because he didn't seem to really care too much about my safety or my health, let alone his own. He didn't ask me if I was hurt, if I had any scratches, broken bones or bruises. My body sure as hell felt like a big-ass bruise.

I would lock myself in the bathroom at times, and he would say, "You're the stupidest Mother Fucking Bitch I have ever met in my life. That's why I fuck around with other women, way better than your ugly ass. You don't know how to fuck, you don't know how to suck dick, and you wonder why a nigga cheating."

Twenty minutes later, he expected me to ride him, and have oral sex with him because he said sorry.

Another occasion, he came in drunk and demanded I have sex with him. I wasn't present emotionally, and didn't want him to touch me. He held me down with both hands, started licking me all over my face, and told me to shut the fuck up and take it when I screamed for him to stop. He was out of control, covering my mouth with his hand, mocking me saying stop. He pulled my underwear down, and said, "You're going to give me my pussy." He spit on his hand, and penetrated me. While in his own world, getting his sexual fix, he didn't know I was crying. If he did, he didn't care one bit. I felt powerless, like I could just die. I felt like raw meat, and raw meat has no emotions or soul.

## JUST THE CLOTHES ON MY BACK

I am in peace. I have no fear. I was able to walk away, knowing there's a better life for me than the one I left behind. I could've been arrested or killed last night, but my Father in heaven held me under his wing. He said you are my daughter and I care for you. Live the blessed life that I already have given you. So now I pray for strength to stay away. I am safe with a mind of peace, with just the clothes on my back.

National Domestic Violence Hotline: 1-800-799-7233

Maybe you are still in denial or disbelief, or still doubting yourself. STOP IT! H.E.E.D. THE RED FLAGS! (HATE+ ENVY + ENMITY + DENIAL & DISORIENTATION = DEATH)

## Chapter Five

Raymond was proud to be an uncle. His baby sister Carla had her first baby. He invited his sister and niece to stay with us for the weekend. I didn't argue with it, because he had been drinking and I knew how his behavior could be. I tried to convince him to do it another time, due to the fact it was my weekend to work and I had to be up early, but he didn't listen.

I went to go pick up Carla and her newborn baby, Justice, like he asked me to. On the way back to our place, I explained to Carla that it wasn't the fact that I didn't want them to come over, but the reason was because of him drinking, and what happens when he drinks. She understood, and knew the only reason she came over in the first place was because he demanded it in his charming way.

When we arrived, Raymond was waiting for us. He asked me to help her get situated. He started to set up the playpen, but couldn't get it assembled correctly. I suggested something about how he should do it, but I got belittled for it.

"Let me see what the fuck you can do, since you know so goddamn much," Raymond said as he left out with his sister and the baby, and headed for the store.

He was surprised when he walked in. I had the playpen set up the right way. The screws just needed to be tightened. He'd already been drinking since the early afternoon, up until late that evening. He cussed me out in front of his sister, grabbed me, and kicked me out the door with his Timberland boots. "Stupid-ass bitch," he said as he slammed the door in my face and locked it.

Why did he do this? My thought was insecurity, jealousy, envy, or maybe because I made a smart comment. I started to think it was my fault and I deserved it.

I heard Carla scream, "Raymond, don't do that!"

I banged on the door, but he wouldn't let me in. Somehow I managed to get my keys before he threw me out of my own residence. I drove to the nearest gas station up the street.

"Sir, could you please call the police, my husband is drunk, and he threw me out of our apartment." The gas station attendant saw I was hysterical and called the police in an instant. He repeated my name over the phone to 911.

"Ma'am, wait right here, the police are going to meet you here at the gas station."

"Thank you."

"No problem."

The last time I remember him kicking me was when I was lying on the floor, and he was sitting on the couch drinking a fifth of Hennessey. He kept asking me why I wouldn't just divorce him. I simply ignored his question. He got mad and kicked me in the stomach with his Timberland boots then too, because I wouldn't say anything to him.

When the officer showed up, I explained to him what had happened. He said that he would follow me to the apartment. I told the officer I just wanted to get my things and leave. When I and Officer Mike arrived, he asked Raymond to explain his side of the story. Raymond claimed that I got mad over something stupid, and I just started yelling and screaming for no reason. He didn't say why I yelled and screamed. Officer Mike said one of us had to leave, or both of us would go to jail. Officer Mike's partner saw that we had called the cops to this address on three previous occasions in the past. They were very close to taking both of us to jail. Yes, the both of us. I called the police and Raymond called the police. I showed the police my bruises, and Raymond showed the scratches I put on him. That must have been comic relief for them.

"I'm just going to stay here until she gets all of her things," Officer Mike stated to Raymond.

I decided to get all my clothes and belongings so I wouldn't have to return for any reason. Raymond tried to make it appear and sound like I was crazy. I was just crazy for letting him back into my life.

"Yeah, go ahead and run, just like you always do. I hope you got everything, too. I'm tired of kissing your ass."

I drove away. My car was packed to the top, and I had no idea where I was going. I was too embarrassed to go to any of my family. I called my mother-in-law, Miss Chapman, his mother. I exhaled after she said she would be looking out for me. I put a comforter over my clothes, especially the stereo I had in the back seat, until the morning. I ended up calling into work, being that I didn't want to go into work bruised, was worn out, and had to be to work in less than four hours. I hadn't had a night so peaceful in a long time. I was always walking on eggshells at home with Raymond.

The landlord started to call my mother's house to get his rent money, but I ignored him at first, because I felt betrayed. Raymond was still there, and I knew he was ignoring the landlord too. What made me give in was that Aaron's Rental started calling for their money, or else they were going to report the furniture we rented as stolen, and the contract was in my name. Raymond must have disappeared, because they said they had made several attempts to pick up the furniture, but they never got an answer. So, I finally got in touch with the landlord, and told him I needed to get the furniture out of the apartment.

*Perpetuality*

"I want to give you your furniture, but you haven't made an attempt to pay your rent. Your rent is $500, and that's what you agreed to."

I explained the situation about Raymond and me. He settled for $250. My mom and stepdad drove me over to pay the landlord. The landlord and I made amends with each other and got an understanding. He didn't know what was going on when he didn't hear from me or Raymond, and the last time he visited the apartment, Raymond had left it a total mess, like he had a party or something. He said there were beer bottles and trash everywhere.

"You can call Aaron's and have them pick up the furniture as soon as possible."

"Thank you."

About a month or so later, I filed for a divorce with Legal Aide. Raymond was served the papers while he was in jail, where they kept him for about 2-3 weeks for driving with a suspended license. To be totally honest with you, I'd lost count on how many times we had separated at this point. I get dizzy sometimes just thinking about it.

\* \* \*

I had gone back to Raymond again. I didn't go through with the divorce. One night, after a revival at All Praises Church of God in Christ (C.O.G.I.C), I gave his brother Lucas a ride home. Lucas was playing the organ for the church that night. When I pulled up in front of the high rise, guess who was standing there? Raymond. He'd been staying with his cousin Gary.

It wasn't by happenstance that he'd been out there, or so I thought. I hadn't seen any of them in about five months. I was happy to see him. He asked me to pick him up in the morning, after he said he missed me, loved me, and asked me how I was doing in school. I was taking summer courses at Monroe Community College. I knew it was too soon to go back to him, but I didn't want to be lonely, and I missed him, and I loved him. I was in the process of getting another apartment in the city, on Arnett Boulevard, close to Genesee Street. I stayed upstairs over a storefront.

We moved into the apartment. I paid the security deposit and first month's rent. We both signed the lease. I took him to Legal Aide with me to sign for the divorce to be stopped. I felt in my stomach I shouldn't have signed it, but I was still hoping for the better. I had called Bobby the car salesman to let him know I was going back to Raymond. I had been seeing Bobby off and on intimately.

"I hope the best for you. He had you first. You know my number if you need me."

"Thank you." A part of me regretted I had to tell Bobby I was not going to see him anymore, because he showed me love and really cared about me.

Raymond was still always late picking me up from work. I would get off at 11:00 p.m., and he'd come at 11:45 or later with the car I payed for. There was always an excuse. One night when he came to pick me up, he was drunk, and his cousin Gary was in the back seat. When I got in the car, he knew I was going to say something about him driving while being drunk, and without a license. He said his cousin Sean had got into some beef and was shot. His cousin Gary was backing him up. They were telling the story of how everything went down. I wanted to believe it, but I didn't. I humbled myself and said I was sorry, and asked was he okay. When we got to the apartment, he wanted to drop me off and keep going. I asked, "Why are you dropping me off? I'll go with you to the hospital. You don't need to be driving anyway."

*Perpetuality*

"Gary can drive then," He said in an angry tone.

"Hell no. What hospital are you going to?"

"Rochester General, you stupid-ass bitch." He was filled with rage and hate. He started to attack me as Gary held him back from taking another hit or jumping on me. I found it weird that he didn't want me to go to the hospital with him. He said his cousin was in the ICU. I don't remember what time he came home that night, but I didn't have control over my own car.

The next day, he stopped by the drugstore to pick up a get-well card for his cousin. I signed the card to go along with the game he was playing. When we arrived at the hospital, he asked me if I wanted to come in. He played it off all the while. When we got to the ICU, he asked me to stay in the waiting area, because only a certain number of people could go back, which I already knew, but when he went through the double doors and I was left out, either it was another woman or there wasn't a cousin named Sean who was shot the night before.

One night Raymond had been drinking, and he got mad because I wouldn't give him my car keys. I ran and locked myself in the bathroom and took my cell phone with me as I called 911. He started to bang on the door, and his banging led to him kicking the door in. I screamed, and as he was trying to kill me with his bare hands, I just knew this night would be the end of my life. When he realized the police were on their way, he ran and escaped through the bedroom window. When the police got there, they asked where he was. I told them he left through the window. I told them he had been drinking.

"Do you want to go to the hospital?"

"No."

"Do you want to press charges?"

"No."

This isn't the first time he's done this, is it?"

"No."

"And you went back to him?"

"I thought he would change."

"Young lady, I know you love your husband, but these are red flags. This is not what love is."

I nodded my head, agreeing with him, but at the same time I didn't want to hear what he had to say, even though I felt like shit, even though my lip was swollen and I almost had my teeth knocked out, even though I was bruised all over, banged up, bloody here and there. I didn't realize how bad I looked until I forced myself to look in the mirror before I got in the shower.

I ended up leaving this apartment too, because Raymond wouldn't. I went to go stay with my mother. I stayed long enough to save money for another apartment not too far from Monroe Community College, where I was attending full-time. One morning, I got a call from Raymond's mother saying that he was admitted to the hospital and had been there for a week. She said he had been having problems with his heart. I wanted to jump in my car right away and get to his side, but I couldn't go. I didn't want to run into or face any of his ex-lovers or any of his side chicks.

A couple of years prior to this, when he was admitted for the same problem, I was surprised by his ex-girlfriend Shauna sitting by his bedside after coming back from freshening up at home. So I chose not to go, but prayed that he was going to be okay. I felt guilty and called the hospital and spoke to his nurse. She said that he was doing better, and that he was going to be okay.

A couple of months later, I called Raymond's mother to give him my phone number so he could call me. After talking to him on the phone a couple of times, after him crying crocodile tears and giving the

## *Perpetuality*

"Baby I was wrong and I'm going to do better, I promise," speech, come to find out we were minutes from each other. He had been staying with a guy friend. He bought me a dozen red roses and we went out to eat at Red Lobster, and I invited him over after. We made passionate love after he romanced me and shed tears over how much he loved, missed, and needed me. It was a wrap. We were back together again. I couldn't wait, anyway, to make love on my new queen-sized bed, and show him my new bedroom suite.

After the honeymoon phase was over, I knew I was going through hell again, except a hotter temperature. I put up with him staying out all times of night, and he started drinking heavily again while driving my car, the same one we both were almost killed in. The same car I had to pay $900 for the body work to be fixed (which could've been much more, but my stepdad Melvin knew someone who could do it cheaper). That car was never the same.

I trusted, prayed, and believed Raymond would stop drinking and driving, that he would stop lying, stop making me feel less of a woman. We moved from the upstairs apartment to the downstairs apartment because he thought it looked better, because it was remodeled. I didn't want to move. I was tired of moving, and I wanted to stay and liked the upstairs apartment, the one I paid for and chose. This time around I was starting to speak up more, not being passive, not being afraid to tell him like it was in a loving way, trying my best not to put him down. I encouraged him, told him, asked him to stop drinking and driving.

The first time he got pulled over, the officer gave him a warning. He was arrested after two more strikes. Yes, within a month's time he had gotten three DUIs. I was taking a class in the evening. Raymond was on his way to pick me up in my car. After sitting and waiting, I walked out to the car as he pulled up. Then I saw two Sheriff cars pull up behind him. I was so fucking embarrassed. Yes, right in front of the college. I was praying that we weren't seen by someone we knew.

"Do you know why I'm pulling you over, Sir?"

"I know I was going pretty fast. I was picking my wife up here."

"You were doing 65 in a 45-mph zone."

I could tell by looking and listening to him he had been drinking. I knew the Sheriffs were going to give him a DUI test. They asked him to step out the car. He messed up on walking the straight line. He was arrested, and was trying to tell me something from the back seat of the police car. I really wasn't trying to hear it. I was more bothered by the fact that his cousin Gary was in the passenger seat.

I dropped his cousin off home. I didn't have much to say. I was in another zone, just wanted to go home. My car was a mess. Cigarette burns and ashes everywhere, sticky spots here and there from beer and liquor. When I arrived home, it was about 11 p.m. I ate the hot wings and fries he had left in the car. I was praying and hoping he was okay. Even though I felt a burden lifted when he was gone, I missed him.

I answered the telephone.

"Baby?"

"Hey."

"The officer wants to speak to you so he can confirm my address."

"Hello Mrs. Wilson. I just need to confirm your husband's address. Are you his wife?"

"Yes."

"What is your address?"

"549 Linden Street, Rochester, New York, 14620."

"Okay, Mrs. Wilson, I'm going to release him over to you."

"Thank you, Officer." I was in shock. I couldn't believe it. All I could say was, thank you Jesus for the favor.

*Perpetuality*

The officer flashed his bright light when they arrived. I came downstairs and the officer released Raymond.

"Hey, Boo Boo," Raymond said with a big grin and kiss.

When we went inside I gave him another kiss and hug. He had an arrogant and egotistical attitude. Like it was because of his doing he was released, when it was really God.

Another night, he went out and took the car. He was dressed up in a sweat suit outfit with his Timberlands that I bought for him. He was supposed to bring back a sandwich from Subway before he went to do his thing. A couple of hours went by, and I received a phone call between twelve and one o'clock in the morning. It was him saying that he had been arrested, and that he was coming by in a cop car. The officer was going to let him give me my car keys, his cell phone, and money he had.

Grandma was not going to bail him out this time. He was going to have to serve his time. Before the officer took Raymond away, he asked me to call his cousin Lorenzo and his wife Sabrina to take me to find my car, where he had parked it. It was about two o'clock in the morning when I called them and let them know Raymond had been arrested for driving under the influence, and was caught without a driver's license. Raymond told me that he parked the car in one of his friends' driveway, somewhere off of Troup and Reynolds Street. I was praying my car was okay, and that nothing had happened to it. Lorenzo and Sabrina picked me up, and we drove around the neighborhood, looking for my red Plymouth Neon, but we couldn't find it. We circled around and around, looking for about a half hour. I thought that the officer decided to have it towed, but I knew Raymond had told me that the officer let him park it in a driveway.

I went to the police station for the area where he had been arrested, and asked to get in touch with the officer that had arrested

Raymond. They didn't have any information that my car had been towed, so they asked me to wait for Officer Mendez's call. He called me in the afternoon the next day. He was very pleasant. He gave me specific directions to where I could find my car. Raymond was drunk that night, and what he had told me was a different story.

It was a pleasant day to walk, so that's what I did. None of my family members knew what had happened. I didn't want to bother asking them to take me to get my car, and not only that, I didn't want to hear what they had to say about the situation, even though I already knew it was fucked up. I prayed and asked God to go before me. I was walking on street corners I preferred not to walk on, but I knew the Holy Spirit was my guide, and was praying the blood of Jesus at the same time. I didn't take my purse, just my ID, keys, and about $8 in cash. Praise the Lord, there it was. After walking from one side of town to another, walking on Upper Falls Boulevard, I ended up on a side street, off of Joseph Avenue. The car was dirty inside and out. When I got inside the car, it smelled like cigarettes and liquor. The gas tank was on empty, but I was able to make it to the nearest gas station.

For the next week or so, I contemplated what I should do about the apartment with Raymond and the car. Raymond told me he didn't want me to be alone. We were behind in rent and the car payments. I ended up giving up the apartment and decided to let the Plymouth Neon get repossessed at my mother's house. He suggested I go stay with his mother, Miss Chapman, and save some money until he got out of jail, and then we would move to Atlanta. I even withdrew from the nursing program at Monroe Community College. I focused on working as many hours as I could so we could leave Rochester. I was known as the double queen. I worked sixteen-hour shifts back to back as a Certified Nursing Assistant. I remember working 104+ hours in a two-week pay period, sometimes more. I always made sure he had commissary, faithfully. I spent hundreds of dollars on the collect calls so he could call anytime he wanted to. I went to visit him twice a week. Sometimes I didn't know what to say. I didn't have much to say. He would fuss at me sometimes because he said I was too quiet. One visit, he embarrassed me by getting loud and belittling me in front of everybody. I ended up leaving as I burst into tears. It took everything I had in me to hold it together until I left the visiting area. I didn't understand how he could allow himself to be so cruel to me after all I had done for him, and for us.

Sometimes I felt like I was being brainwashed, lost in a trance. He confessed to sleeping with a couple of women while we were together. One of them being the white girl he sold the blue Honda to, or to her father, rather. He claimed he saw her when he went out one night, and he slept with her while her dad was at work. He also admitted to sleeping with the young lady who would come over with her boyfriend. His name was Raymond also. He told me I was at work, and he slept with her while her boyfriend was passed out drunk, upstairs in our house we rented on Priscilla Street. He also admitted having oral sex with one of the strippers I knew. Yes, I compromised to go to the strip clubs with Raymond because I thought, or he made me believe, we would have a better, open, romantic, and exciting marriage. On more than a couple of occasions I engaged in ménage à trois, one of them being with Tammy. He convinced me one night after giving me oral sex, and while fucking me, he asked me was I sure that I loved him. He brought up Tammy and how she told him I was sexy and had a nice body. He asked me would I have a trois, and would I do it for him as he fucked me harder and harder. I gave in and said yes.

Raymond drove us to a club in Buffalo from Rochester. One night, in lake effect snow, the visibility was bad. Talk about awkward, but the Hennessey and the smoke warmed me up to get comfortable with the situation. After sharing my man at the club, I shared him and myself sexually at a hotel we all went to after. I started to get comfortable and enjoy it until I started to feel some type of way when I felt like there was a competition about who could suck and deep throat his dick better and fuck him better or take dick better, in whatever position he demanded. He mostly enjoyed watching us please each other with the dildos and giving each other oral sex, giving us instructions, telling us what to do and vice versa. Come the next morning, I asked myself, *Did this really just happen?* Especially after fighting this woman in our townhouse a year or so prior. Ain't that a bitch. Yes, I would say I was definitely brainwashed, or under a mojo spell or something. We dropped Tammy off home, and I don't think I made it to church that Sunday.

I was heartbroken when he told me he had slept with these women, which I didn't know he had. I cried and cried, and couldn't understand. I still wanted to support him, even after his confession.

I started making preparations in September to move to Atlanta. I would put him on three-way during a lot of the business calls. I was able to get a P.O. Box and opened a bank account at Wachovia at the time, from Rochester. Rochester didn't even have a Wachovia bank. I got us approved for an apartment in Dunwoody, Sandy Springs. That was truly God, because I had owed an apartment on my credit.

His release date was on a Monday in November, but I had written a letter of request to let him out the Friday before, at midnight. I rented a Ford Focus from Budget Rent-a-Car. It was over $600 for three weeks. We were going to be in Atlanta for two. I had saved over $3,000 in the bank to take care of our business. I was excited that he was coming home that night. I wanted to do something special. I just couldn't imagine going straight to his Mother's house after him being released. I honestly wanted him all to myself before anybody got to see him. I rented a hotel room with a jacuzzi, and mirrors on the ceiling above the bed. I wanted this night to be so special. I had the aromatherapy candles, my red lingerie outfit. I filled the Jacuzzi with bubble bath, floating candles, and pink and red rose petals.

It was getting near midnight, the time I had to arrive to pick him up. I got so caught up in the moment while decorating the room that it was too late to order take out. I couldn't be late. I was going to surprise him with just my skimpy red lingerie under my trench coat, my long blonde hair, and stilettos. I was really feeling myself; I thought the way I looked, this man could wait for dinner, and he could eat me instead.

When I pulled up in front of the jail, I had 10-15 minutes before he walked out. Words can't explain what I was feeling. I played some slow jams, thinking it would help set the mood. There Raymond was, walking out with two bags in his hand. I remembered he had the same outfit on he had got arrested in, except he had gained weight. He was really buff and it looked good on him. I imagined myself getting out of the car, running into his arms, sticking my tongue down his throat, and seducing him with the sexy surprise I had under my coat, but it didn't happen that way.

"Aren't you going to pop the trunk?"

I sat in the driver's seat the whole time. I was disappointed in myself and felt guilty that I didn't seize the moment. When he got in the car, our vibes were not hitting like they should. We ended up at Tim Horton's to get a couple of sandwiches. I was driving a route he didn't expect, which was back to the hotel.

"Where are you going?" he said with an attitude.

"I can't tell you right now."

He demanded that I take him to his mother's house. I knew we had to go back to the hotel, even if I went by myself, because I had left the candles burning. That's exactly how my heart felt—like it was burning. I was hurt and disappointed that he didn't want to even see where I wanted to take him.

When we arrived, his mother was so excited to see him, and about twenty minutes into the visit, I demanded that we leave after he decided he just wanted to lie down and read his Holy Bible. His Mother encouraged him to go with me. After all, I was his wife.

He was surprised to see how the room looked. I was thankful that the burning candles were okay. Except the floating candles in the Jacuzzi had burned out, some melted. After talking about our plans to head to Atlanta and his time spent in jail, while sipping on some White Zinfandel, he took his sweatshirt off. I was shocked to see how big he was. I knew he weighed at least 200 pounds. He was solid and buff all over, but I realized muscles and good looks don't make a man. I knew from what I had experienced that night, not too much had changed. He wanted me to copy and do everything in the many porno flicks I purchased at the hotel. I had spent money on clothes and Timberland boots. We stayed in hotels for the next four to five days until we left for Atlanta. I knew I was going for another rollercoaster ride when he said he was taking the car to go holler at his boys. He left about nine or ten at night, and didn't return until six or seven the next morning. The bad part is that he shouldn't have been driving, he had no license, it was suspended, but he didn't care, and I compromised and went along with it.

## Chapter Six

We were off to Atlanta. I can't remember what day of the week it was, but we arrived days before Thanksgiving. We stayed with his cousin Mitch and his wife Leah, and their two young boys, Darwin and Daniel. I was so happy to be in Atlanta. Words can't explain what I felt when I arrived. It felt like home, where I was supposed to be.

We came in town with about $2500, and I'm sad to say I don't even know where it all went to. Well, yes I do. Most of the money was to go on the apartment, pay a couple of months ahead, furniture and utilities. We stayed in Atlanta a little over two weeks. The first night we went out to party. We spent money like it was water. I worked hard, so damn hard to save this money. Raymond called himself handling the money. Even though I was having fun, when I did speak up about how out-of-control this was getting, he would say not to worry about it. That I should learn how to enjoy myself, because I had worked so hard, but at the same time he was manipulating me so he could drink and do what he wanted to do regardless of our priorities and responsibilities. We were eating out just about every day, drinking some kind of liquor every day, Long Islands, Hennessey, Heineken, you name it, including the hundreds of dollars going to Magic City, throwing money to strippers, table and lap dances, and going to other strip joints and drinking.

Our application and deposit had already been paid for the apartment. It was in a nice area, in Sandy Springs. They held the apartment for us until we returned in January. We didn't do anything we were supposed to do with the money saved. We had to work and save money when we got back to Rochester. The whole eight months he was away, I had stayed with his mother and paid rent to her faithfully. Before we left to go to Atlanta, I wanted to pay her for December's rent, and I very well could have, but I let him talk me into paying her when we got back from Atlanta.

We arrived in Rochester around the 8th of December of 2003. All our money was spent, and I didn't have Miss Chapman's rent money. Rent was only $250. His mother wasn't a fool and knew there was no reason for the rent not being paid. I don't think it was two weeks late when she showed us how serious she was. She called Raymond and I to come in the living room one morning while we were sleeping. There were two police officers confirming that she wanted us to leave if she didn't have any rent from us by the end of the week. Raymond was furious that his own mother called the police, and I was surprised, but no matter how furious or surprised we were, honestly, when it came down to it, I should have kept my word. But now that Raymond and I were together, things had changed. My behavior changed, my confidence and attitude too. His grandparents, Mr. and Mrs. Perry, let us stay with them until we made our final move to Atlanta.

Everything he said to me about being faithful and being a better man for God, me, and us, went straight down the toilet. It was a Sunday morning, and I was on my way to church. Just as I was about to put the key into the ignition, I noticed a card and letter in the door, on the driver's side. I was so fucking pissed. It was an *I love you* card and letter from Selena, who I thought was his so-called home girl, and just a friend. I ran back into the house and upstairs to wake him up. I questioned him about what she said about them being made for each other, and that she was in love with him, and she even mentioned them kissing. Of course he told me what I wanted to hear, even though it was a lie. Raymond said he had to leave her alone. He said nothing could be between them because he was married to me and he loved me. He didn't know she felt that way about him. I knew it was a bunch

## Perpetuality

of bullshit. Raymond had the nerve to tell me to calm down, and that I was getting upset over nothing. I felt betrayed. After eight whole months of being by his side and going to visit him faithfully just about every week. I maybe missed one or two because I was sick. After working sixteen hours a day, accumulating 100 hours and more at times, paying on the phone bill so he could call collect. I made sure he had commissary every two weeks. Thinking about all I went through for him and had sacrificed for this man. I withdrew from the nursing program. After all this flashed before me, I cussed him out like a dog and apologized to Mrs. Perry, his grandmother, who heard the argument down stairs. I left out for church, and still after all that, I still managed to sing in the choir and get my shout on.

I ended up owing Wachovia Bank over $1,000 after we finally turned in the Ford Focus. I was so furious and disappointed in myself. This gave me flashbacks of how my sister Lauren's car was vandalized because she let Raymond drive it a few times. One of his side chicks keyed up my sister's Blue Ford Focus. She spray-painted white writing on the car windows and window shield, "Fuck you liar. Bitch," and a tire or two was slashed. I was in disbelief because I chose to still be with this man, and my family was being affected too.

The last couple of weeks before it was time for us to leave for Atlanta were hell. Raymond was back to drinking heavily, liquor and beer, a lot of it. He started being more emotionally abusive. After he got into it with his grandfather, we definitely had to leave. We had one week. His grandmother gave us the money to go, and she rented the car for us as well.

One weekend before we left I got sick like a dog. While at my Aunt Charmaine's house, I got worse before I got better. My brother Andre, his wife Latesha, and I were spending time with Aunt Charmaine before she moved to Texas. Raymond kept calling me, demanding that

I better come home. It was one or two o'clock in the morning. I tried to explain to him how sick I was, but he wasn't trying to hear it. I could tell by his voice he had been drinking. I had been back and forth to the bathroom so many times with my face in the toilet and sink. I had thought about just camping out there for the rest of the night. My Aunt Charmaine was right there to rub my back and reassure me that I was going to be okay.

My brother Andre and Latesha dropped me off at Raymond's grandparents' house. It was after two o'clock in the morning. I went upstairs to the bedroom and Raymond was passed out from drinking so much. I took a couple of Pepto chewables and tried to go to sleep. I then noticed his phone ringing. I got curious, and started looking up the names he had in his phone. Selena's number was there. She had called him just hours ago. This was the same home girl he said he had to turn loose, the same home girl who wrote the love notes in the card I found in the car. It dawned on me that I had seen her name on the visitor's list for Raymond when I went to go see him.

We headed down south about four o'clock in the morning, in the Ford Taurus his grandmother, Mrs. Perry had rented for us and with the $1,000 she took out a loan for. We made only a few stops.

I was overjoyed when I started to see the red clay. It was in the early evening when we arrived. His cousins Mitch and Leah hadn't gotten home yet, just their two sons, Darwin and Daniel. The next day Mitch followed us to Budget to drop off the rent-a-car. Raymond and I got into a heated argument about his home girl Selena. I don't even remember how the argument started. I know that he admitted to kissing her. I lost it when he told me that. How could he even think about touching another woman, after all the sacrifices I made for him?

We stayed with Mitch and Leah a couple of weeks so we wouldn't have to pay any pro-rated rent. We moved into our apartment around the first of February. Neither one of us had found a job yet. Those couple of weeks we stayed with his cousins, they started to see some true colors. Colors I'm sure they didn't want or expect to see. We went out with them on a few occasions, to Bigelows, Tanqueray, and a karaoke bar across the street from where they lived, where we went almost every week. Mitch and Leah had bought a gallon of E&J. They said a gallon usually lasts them a couple of months, but because Raymond was around, it was gone in less than two weeks.

One late night when he was passed out, I got curious. I knew that he had a recorder on his Nextel, so I decided to check it out. After playing around with the gadgets on the phone, I finally got to listen to a couple of the recordings. It was his home girl Selena. I heard her saying how he made her feel, and that he was just the right size for her, and that she loved him. What's crazy is, I went along as planned to move into our new apartment. I said nothing else about her.

It was Super Bowl Sunday when we moved into our new apartment. There was a sports bar right down the street, within walking distance. We met another couple, Tim and Pam, while playing pool. Raymond always struck up conversations with strangers, always friendly and considerate. We were always complimented on what a beautiful couple we were. Tim was from Baltimore and Pam was from Detroit. They had just relocated to Atlanta as well, and had been dating a couple of months. They were really cool.

We all ended up leaving together and going to another sports bar because there was an altercation between Raymond and a waitress about how much she charged us. After charging us for one price, and we had already paid, she came back telling us she under-quoted us and we owed more money. Raymond already had some drinks in him. I already had a couple of long islands. They called the police. Raymond encouraged them to do so. In the end, they just told us we weren't allowed back in the bar anymore. I was pissed the fuck off, because they kept my driver's license. The protocol was to give them ID to hold the pool table.

We rode in Pam's car to another sports bar, and got more drunk and stupid. Raymond just fell right in with the crowd. I was praying I didn't get sick after having so many margaritas. It started to get really late. We didn't want the night to end. Tim and Pam had to get up for work the next morning, but Raymond had the gift of gab and convinced them to hang a little longer. We ended up driving around Atlanta for almost two hours, then they finally dropped us off home and said goodnight.

Raymond and I were at the Perimeter Mall one day, when Pam and Tim called. They said they were looking for an apartment, and the apartments they had looked at so far didn't interest them at all. So we referred them to Centergate Morgan Falls, now known as the Residences at Morgan Falls, where we were staying. They said they would put in an application. Raymond and I both had filled out applications and faxed off resumes. He had even been on some interviews, which he was very good at.

One day, I decided to check out this school called ACT for medical assistant. Raymond had cussed me out during an argument that morning. He called me on my cell phone, but I didn't answer. It was about seven o'clock in the evening when I got on the northbound train. Pam called me saying Raymond had been worried sick about me, and asked if I was okay. She said they were going to pick me up from the North Springs Station. On my way to the station, I could feel something just wasn't right. Raymond was with Pam and Tim when they pulled up in the station. Raymond got out of the back seat, and he had a 20-ounce Bud Light in his hand. I could tell it wasn't his first one. When he got out the car, he started cussing me out. "What the

*Perpetuality*

fuck is wrong with you, dumb bitch? I swear to God you are so fucking dumb. I can't stand your stupid ass. I've been calling you all fucking day, and you don't fucking answer." He lashed out to hit me, but Tim jumped in front of him and tried to calm him down. Pam was getting frustrated. We all got inside the car.

Even though Pam and Tim were in the front, I felt so scared and alone. I was alone in the back seat with Raymond, and he demanded that I answer his questions about where I'd been, and who I was with, and why it took me so long, because he is my fucking husband. I was afraid to look at him again, because all I saw was evil, and a demonic look in his eyes. Next thing I knew, he punched me in the temple of my forehead, saying, "Stupid-ass bitch." I saw stars and my vision got blurry.

Tim warned him to calm down. I wanted to believe I was having a nightmare, but this was my reality. For some reason I had a flashback to when we lived on Priscilla Street in Rochester, a night he was kneeling and crying at the foot of the bed and had threatened to shoot himself in the head with the .38 revolver handgun. He was sobbing tears, telling me he would kill himself if I left him. I promised him and convinced him that I wasn't going to leave him and he couldn't believe otherwise, because I loved him and nobody else.

When we arrived at our apartment, after what seemed like the longest ride ever, Raymond asked Tim and Pam to come upstairs. After they said no, Raymond said fuck all ya'll, and made his way upstairs, but before he got out of the car, we had started a discussion about God. Raymond started to brag about how I was such a good Christian, and how I could tell them about God, but because I chose not to really partake in the conversation, or the debate, and was still in pain from him punching me in the temple, he told me I was so damn stupid.

After a few minutes, Tim decided to go check on him. "He just has a lot on his mind," Tim said as he got out of the car.

Pam was in shock. "I would've never thought he had this side to him."

I kept saying to myself, "I can't believe this. I can't believe this. I can't go back home. We just moved to a new city, and got our apartment."

Pam and I decided to go upstairs. Raymond started to throw a temper tantrum again when he saw me. He belittled me so bad, I felt like he had crumpled me up like a piece of paper and threw me in the trashcan. He was cussing and carrying on, cracking his knuckles as if he was getting ready to fight me. When he came back inside from being on the balcony, he slammed the door so hard that he cracked the glass.

Before I knew it, he picked up my cell phone and threw it at me, but he missed and hit the wall, and my cell phone broke. Pam had seen and heard enough, and said I could stay the night at their house.

A few hours later, Raymond called me on Pam's phone. He told me he had packed his things and he had his friend Canon schedule him a flight back to Rochester the next morning. I knew he was drunk, and I hoped it was true, but I knew it wasn't, even though he gave me the confirmation number. The next morning, I rode with Tim and Pam. We dropped Pam off to work first. I didn't like the fact that I was left alone with Tim without Pam being around. I didn't want thoughts crossing anybody's head that I was trying to hit on their man, mainly worried about what Raymond would say, think, or do about it.

Tim headed to a temp agency and we were there a long time. When we arrived at my and Raymond's apartment, I was hoping he had left like he said, but I knew he hadn't gone anywhere. When I walked through the door, he totally ignored me and acted like I didn't exist. He had his clothes folded up, but they weren't in a suitcase. I

*Perpetuality*

could hear him talking on the phone in the other room. I could hear clearly he was flirting with another female on the phone about her sexy-ass body. I got angry and cursed him out to his face, and whoever was on the other end could hear me. I dashed out the apartment torn apart. Raymond chased after me, grabbed me, and took me to the bedroom, where we tussled. He held me down and said he was sorry, and that it was my fault. I gave in once again and that was that.

As time went on, I finally got an interview at Beverly Nursing and got hired on the same day. It was for a night position. Raymond didn't want me to commute that late at night, so he demanded that I ask for another shift. I could tell the Nurse Manager was disappointed that I didn't take the position, but she was nice enough to refer me to another Beverly Nursing facility. I got hired for the 7-3 p.m. shift and was required to work three weekends a month. The C.N.A position paid $8.50 an hour, and I had five years of experience. Talk about back breaking. A lot of my experience was in the nursing home, but being from Upstate New York, I was used to getting paid for my labor. You know what I mean? This to me was just straight-up slavery. Taking care of ten patients or more, along with taking vital signs on each patient, and 20-30 minutes of charting on a kiosk for every patient, I was done. Over it.

One morning, I was running late and couldn't find a pay phone to let my job know I was going to be late. Our cell phones were out of service at the time. I arrived a little past 8 a.m. I had a migraine headache so bad that I felt sick to my stomach. I started work after apologizing for being late. I knew I wasn't going to stay the whole shift, and I had signed up to work a double shift. The supervisor came to me while I was taking care of a patient.

"I tried to call you to let you know you didn't need to come in this morning, and that you can just work the 3-11. You need to have a phone so we can reach you."

"Well, my phone isn't in service, and I don't think I'm going to be able to stay too much longer, because I have a bad migraine and I am nauseated."

With a sarcastic attitude, she said I needed to hurry up and take something and get better because I had to stay and work. She sounded too much like a redneck, and she had the nerve to be standing in my face too. I wanted to jump all over that lady's ass, but I gave a smirk and said okay. I finished taking care of my last two patients, and told my partner I was working with what had just happened. She said that she had been wanting to leave for a long time.

After I found out what time my lunch break was, I said, "No disrespect towards you, but when I break, I'm gone, and I'm not coming back." This situation put the icing on the cake. A few days prior, I was left alone with two men, one being over 200 pounds, the other over 300 pounds, for total care and hoyer lifts, and I was supposed to be in orientation. It was after 11 a.m. when I left Beverly Nursing and never looked back, except to pick up my check a week later. I arrived just in time before it was going to be sent in the mail.

Raymond was surprised to see me come home early that day. He was hanging out with Tim, drinking beer and E&J.

"What happened?"

"I quit."

"You fucking lying right? We got rent and bills to pay."

He got angry and cussed me out. He didn't even ask if I was okay or what happened. After seeing him sitting up early in the day drinking with Tim, I didn't care. I'm working like a slave, while he has a party?

He told me I needed to go back and go to work. There was no way in hell I was going to do that. He would just have to fight me. Fuck it.

Pam and Tim got approved and moved into the same complex we stayed in. After almost two weeks of being unemployed, I got a job at a dry cleaners down the street, tagging clothes for $7.50 an hour.

One day while I was at work, Raymond came by my job twice. The first time he was just strolling by on his way to the store. The second time he came inside within a couple of hours and asked for my keys, because he said he had lost his. It did cross my mind as weird, but I didn't think much more about it.

On my way home Raymond and Tim picked me up. Raymond walked me inside the apartment, said a few words, *I love you*, gave me a kiss, and walked out with his Bud Light 20 ounce. I walked into the bedroom and noticed the bed comforter wasn't laid out on the floor. We hadn't gotten a mattress yet. The comforter was covering a pile of clothes, and he had thrown in the closet the shoes that I had outside of the closet before I left for work that day. I said to myself, "No, this can't be happening. I knew it was the Holy Spirit leading me back to the living room. When I looked on the fireplace, our wedding pictures, cards from Valentine's Day, and the teddy bears were gone. The fireplace was empty. I looked at the bar where we'd had wedding pictures sitting up as well. They were gone too. I went into the kitchen, opened one of the drawers, and there were the pictures and cards, hidden.

I decided I wasn't going to say anything right away. I wanted to observe what he was going to do when he got back home. I kept cool and calm, didn't say anything, acted normal as possible, except when we went to bed. He wanted to have sex, and I told his ass straight up, "Hell no."

"That's why I'm going to start fucking other women. There's women that look and fuck way better than you."

I felt like all my other organs were burning from my heart melting like wax.

When the morning came, I checked his pockets. I found a box of condoms. Three came in the box, and one was missing. I looked in the trash, but didn't find a used condom. After I returned from the business office to fax my resumes, Raymond was up and I tore the place apart. I fought him, yelled, screamed, and cried. I was in a rage, very angry, and tormented. The sad thing is, I was addicted to him and the drama. It's like I got an adrenaline rush. His excuse was that he held the condoms for his man so his girl wouldn't find them. He said that he could even get his man to admit that they were his condoms. I knew Raymond could get someone to lie, especially when it came down to playing games. When he got out of the shower and got dressed, he tried to cover his tracks by putting the teddy bears, the cards, and pictures back in place. It then occurred to me why he came to my job twice and asked for my keys. He wanted to make sure I was in place so he could do his dirt.

I was always giving him money. More than I kept for myself. Enabling his cigarette and alcohol addictions. He asked me for twenty dollars to fill out an application at the Post Apartments down the street, the same day he asked for my keys. I called the complex that he said he went to submit the application and pay the fee of $20. They didn't have the information on file, and this was the only Post Apartments on Roswell Road.

We were facing eviction at the time, and I lost my job at the cleaners for being late a few times trying to find help for the eviction.

We made arrangements to vacate the apartment, especially after we showed up late to court for the judgement against us. Tim and Pam didn't come around much anymore. They got tired of the drama that was going on all the time. Caesar, Raymond's friend that he met in our complex, helped move us back to Mitch and Leah's place. Raymond and Caesar were going off to Cocoa Beach to sell coach bags. I was speechless. I didn't feel like protesting it. I didn't care if he went or not.

One early morning, I got up and went to this furniture store where I found out some time ago that the owners file divorces. Kirk, the manager, and his wife Kayla were an odd-looking couple. Kirk was white, tall and skinny, and looked like he was in his 60s. His wife Kayla had to be in her early 40s. They directed me to a lady named Stella. I talked to Stella over the phone and told her I wanted a divorce. She charged me $350. She let me put down a deposit of $150, which was just about my last check from the cleaners. Stella was on her way to come get me from the furniture store to start the process.

Stella and her brother picked me up and took me to cash my check. While riding, I gave her a quick history about me and Raymond, and what led up to me wanting a divorce. She suggested that I file a contestant divorce and that it would take one to two months after I have it publicized. I told her I was living with Raymond at his cousin's house. She said it was in my best interest that I move. She offered me to rent a room out of her house for $400 a month. I explained to her that I had just lost my job, and I was planning to move back to Rochester, New York. Stella told me I needed to remain in Georgia until the divorce was final. I told her I would be in touch when they dropped me off at Indian Creek Station.

I arrived back home in the early afternoon. Raymond was sitting on the stairs. I acted calm and pleasant. I told him he was out cold, and I tried to wake him up. I lied and said I had been out window shopping.

The next day he left for Cocoa Beach with Caesar. He was going to be gone for a week. I knew he was going to do a whole lot more than sell Coach bags. The night before, I felt like mud being stepped into when he rolled over after he got his nuts off. I wept while he was thrusting me, and he didn't realize the pain I was in. I didn't have the strength to fight because I had none. When he called me to let me know he had arrived in Cocoa Beach, I called my mom right away. She bought me a plane ticket to leave for Rochester the next morning.

*Perpetuality*

## I CAN BREATHE

No more gritting my teeth, unconsciously stressed. Scared of the one I love, and constantly in distress. Can I breathe? Oh, there's a breath. I forgot I could breathe, my shoulders always raised, intense. The only way I find time to breathe is when I'm not with him, who is now my ex. I can breathe.

National Domestic Violence Hotline: 1-800-799-7233

Maybe you are still in denial or disbelief, or still doubting yourself. STOP IT! H.E.E.D. THE RED FLAGS! (HATE+ ENVY + ENMITY + DENIAL & DISORIENTATION = DEATH)

## Chapter Seven

It was near the end of April 2004 when I landed back in Rochester, New York. I was able to get my job back at Edna Tina Living Center as a C.N.A., and was back on payroll the next week. I knew I wasn't going to stay in Rochester too much longer. I was too ready to head back to Atlanta. That June was the first year of MegaFest, and I was going to be back in Atlanta by then. I purchased my $84 ticket about three weeks in advance. That's just about how much time I gave my family to let them know I was going back to Atlanta. I didn't know where I was going to live. I was trying to get an apartment, but couldn't get approved.

One evening I was in the living room with my mother watching a Lifetime movie. She was happy to hear from whoever was on the other line when she answered the phone.

"Well, you called just in time because she's talking about going back down there in a couple of weeks. It's Leah," my mom whispered to me.

I'm like *okay, why is she sounding so astonished?*

"Okay, I'll let you speak to her."

"Hey Leah."

"Hey girl, how are you?"

"I'm doing good. How are you doing?"

"Good, good. I was just telling your mom that we have the other bedroom furnished, and Raymond isn't staying here anymore. I was calling to see if you might be interested. Mitch and I will work with you until you get on your feet. You know we told you we would love to have you anytime."

"Oh my God. Thank you, thank you, thank you." I was so overjoyed and excited I didn't know what to do with myself.

"So yeah, you let us know when you're coming so we can make arrangements."

"Okay, Leah. I will be coming on the 21st because I'm going to the MegaFest."

"All right, we'll see you then."

I arrived back in Atlanta in the early evening. Mitch and Leah picked me up from Dunwoody Train Station. We didn't discuss anything about Raymond, even though I was anxious to know where he was and who he was with. We were all happy to see each other and I told them I had a nice and safe flight. I was happy to be back in Atlanta. The bedroom was fixed up very nice, and they were only going to charge me $150 a month. They would work with me until I got a job and got on my feet.

They had kept a lot of our things in the closet from when Raymond and I got evicted. I found two pretty Louis Vuitton purses, a cocoa beach key chain, and a pink short outfit. I thought, *how sweet.*

After job hunting one day, I informed Leah that I had an interview at 9:30 in the morning, at Burger King. I thought she had seen a ghost by the look on her face.

"Allana, I didn't want to tell you this, but now I have to. Raymond's been seeing a young lady that works there. He's brought her by here for us to meet her and everything. I tried to talk to him and remind him he's still married, but that's his life. I'm sorry, I didn't want to get caught up between the two of you, but if I was in your shoes, I would want someone to tell me."

"Thank you for telling me, Leah. It's not your fault."

To be honest, I was disappointed, jealous, and embarrassed at the same time.

About a week later, the day after the Fourth of July, the telephone rang while I was doing my hair. I let it keep ringing until it stopped. Less than a minute later, it rang again. It was something about the second time. I ran to go look at the caller ID. It said Savannah Suites.

"Hello?" I said hesitantly.

"Hello."

It was Raymond on the other end.

"How are you?"

"I'm good. How are you?" I said, trying not to sound too happy, even though I was bursting with excitement.

"I miss you."

"I miss you too."

"Listen, let me be honest with you. When you left I did start seeing somebody, but I cut if off when I found out you were back in town. Her name is Taneka, and we were going together for about two months."

I thought to myself, *Boy, he sure didn't waste any time.*

"She knew that I was still in love with you. I told her I knew you had come back to Atlanta. I felt it so strong, we drove to Mitch and Leah's, and I was looking for a car with New York license plates, but didn't see anything. Then I looked up at the bedroom window, and there I saw you, looking through the opened blinds. We drove off in a hurry because I didn't want you to see us."

"So that was ya'll in the black car I saw dash off? I thought something was strange about that. I couldn't see who it was, but I knew there were two people in a sports car."

"You saw that?"

"I sure did."

*Perpetuality*

"Yeah, it was a 2004 Mustang," he said chuckling, in a bragging tone. I didn't care, because in my mind at the time, I was just satisfied with him coming back to me.

I gave Leah a heads-up when she got home and told her I had talked to Raymond and that he was coming by to get me. Raymond was not welcome back at their place, because they let him borrow their Jeep on Memorial Day, about five o'clock in the evening to go pick up a few plates from a barbeque really quick and then come back. Raymond didn't contact Leah or Mitch until hours later, saying that he had drunk too much and didn't want to drive until he got sober. They didn't see Raymond until five o'clock the next morning, and their Jeep was returned smelling like alcohol and cigarettes.

I told Leah that Raymond and I were getting back together, and that I wasn't going to be staying much longer. Leah didn't agree with the decision I had made, but I didn't care. I had my mind made up, and I didn't care what she had to say about it. The next day, Raymond and I rented a room in Doraville at the USA Economy Lodge. We barely had the money to get a room. His grandmother, Mrs. Perry, came to the rescue once again, and sent money Western Union, which paid for our room about two weeks. So much happened in the little time we were at the hotel. One night, before Raymond left out, he brought back a couple of hotdogs with everything on it from the QT gas station next door, a truck stop.

"I'll be back, Boo Boo. I'm going to meet up with Cash to get some drinks. I love you."

"Love you, too."

It was raining cats and dogs that night. Not too long after he left out the door, I got the urge to pray. I was lying prostrate on the floor and began to speak in my prayer language. I started to cry aloud from my gut. I didn't understand at the time why I was weeping so much. This was between twelve and one o'clock in the morning.

    The next day, Raymond wanted to have a barbeque. We got acquainted with some of the neighbors at the hotel, Skye and Mookie, along with a few others. We didn't start the barbeque until 8 or 9 o'clock. I really didn't want to have the barbeque, but Raymond insisted. I came out of the hotel room and noticed him flirting his ass off with one of our neighbors, Lillie, getting into her blue Jeep. I ran up to the Jeep and opened it like I was about to take the door off.

    "Get your motherfucking ass out." I was looking like I wish a bitch would say something.

    I walked my pissed and disappointed ass back to the room. The phone began to ring. I wasn't in the mood to talk to anybody, but I decided to answer it anyway.

    "Hello?"

    "Hey Allana, how are you?"

    "Hey Mitch, how are you doing," I said, trying to sound nice.

    "I'm good. Hey, is Raymond there?" he said hesitantly.

    "Yeah, he's here. Hold on just a minute."

    "Okay, thank you."

    As I walked away from the phone, I was surprised it was Mitch, because he didn't want to have anything to do with Raymond. I walked outside to see where Raymond was. It wasn't hard to find him, because he was always the center of attention, talking loud, laughing, joking, cussing, and carrying on.

    "Raymond, Mitch is on the phone."

    "Mitch? My cousin Mitch?"

    "Yeah, he wants to talk to you."

    The look on Raymond's face told me what I looked like when I answered the phone.

"Hello? Hey, Mitch. What's up, man?"

I was anxious to know what Mitch was saying.

"Nooo. What? Oh my God!"

Raymond dropped the phone as he started to break down and cry.

"Raymond, what's wrong? What happened?"

My first thought was something happened to his grandmother, Mrs. Perry. I tried to console him but he wouldn't let me. He ran out the door. I picked up the receiver of the phone.

"Hello, Mitch. What happened?"

Mitch gave a huge sigh. "Taneka, the young lady Raymond was seeing when you guys separated, was killed last night. You know it was raining last night, right?"

"Oh my God! Yes."

"Well, she pulled over on the highway to help somebody and got hit by a car."

I can't even explain or put into words the shock I was in. There was dead silence that seemed to last forever.

I was very sorry to hear this. I ran outside to see where Raymond was. Everyone at the barbeque wanted to know what the hell was going on.

"He just got a ride with somebody," Mookie said.

Taneka's family stayed in the same apartment complex as Leah and Mitch.

Sheila knocked on my room door. Sheila and her boyfriend, who we had just met a few days prior, stayed on the fourth floor above us.

"Are you okay?"

"Yes. I'll be all right."

"I need to tell you something. Raymond came to my room last night to use the phone. I thought it was weird that he didn't use the phone in his room. He had told me not to tell you, but he was calling

Taneka to see why she was taking so long to come to him, but she never answered the phone. He had walked out to the front of the hotel a couple of times to see if she had showed up, but when he made the last call to her and she didn't answer, he gave up. She was on her way here to see him."

I had no words to speak, no feelings to express. I must have gone into a zone, because she kept asking me if I was okay.

"Yes, I am okay. Thank you for telling me. I know you didn't have to do that."

"Girl, I would've wanted somebody to tell me. I don't know how you do it. You're a strong woman. He doesn't deserve you. I mean, I can't believe he left like that. And you are his wife. Are you sure you don't want any company?"

"No, I'll be all right."

"You want to come upstairs? Craig is gone."

"No. I really need some time alone."

"Okay. Call if you need me."

I appreciated the fact that Sheila came out and told me the truth, and that she was concerned about me. I had only known her for a couple of days. I was in the bed quietly for hours. No television, no music. Nothing.

There was awkward silence between Raymond and I for a few days, and when he did talk to me, he confessed that Taneka had been three months pregnant with his baby. He told me that Taneka's mother didn't want to see him or be bothered when he tried to reach out. He kept blaming himself and saying it was his fault, because she was on her way to see him. Not only that, but she had learned from him to pull over and help people. Raymond did that a lot of times. He was always stopping more than not, to help someone that was stranded. I kept trying to convince him that it wasn't his fault. I even encouraged him to go to the funeral, but at the same time, didn't know if it was such a good idea.

When that Saturday morning came, I asked him if he was sure he didn't want to attend. He kept in touch with one of her cousins. He told me that she was holding their three-month fetus in the coffin. While trying to console him, I felt fucked up at the same time. I got flashbacks when he would tell me something was wrong with me because I never got pregnant. He acted as if he didn't want to be bothered with me or touch me.

We were still struggling week to week, trying to keep a room. Raymond would work at Labor Ready and a moving company when they had work available, or when he did decide to go to work. Skye and Mookie had let us stay in their room one night and we stayed another night at Lillie's and her girlfriend's room—yes the female I caught him flirting with at the barbeque. To say I was embarrassed was an understatement. I swallowed my pride and rolled with it. I never really went to sleep, because they kept the air conditioning on full blast the whole night. Although I was grateful we weren't on the streets, it literally felt like a freezer.

*Lord you're all I need*, is a song I wrote one night after being locked out of our room. It was about ten o'clock at night. I didn't have a cell phone. Nobody I knew was home at the time. There were a couple of men that noticed I was locked out, and would ask me if I was okay. It was hours before Raymond made it back home.

One night, Raymond and I were invited by Jamal and a few others to go to a sports bar down the street from USA Economy Lodge. Jamal was dark-skinned, in his early thirties. While I was sitting at the table, I started to wonder why Raymond was gone so long. Jamal came back from the bar with a couple of more drinks, and told me, "Sweetheart, you need to go check your man. I think he's had too much to drink. He's over there by the games."

I had already had a few long islands myself. Raymond always convinced me that I needed to drink with him in order to have a good time, and that I shouldn't be so damn boring. As I walked up, I saw him flirting and all with a light-skinned female who was wearing sunglasses. His back was facing me, so he didn't see me coming. I slapped him hard on the right side of his head with my right hand. My hand was on fire.

"Nigga, what the hell you think you doing?"

"What the fuck is wrong with you?"

Raymond turned red in the face. He took his glass and threw it at me, grabbed me tightly by both arms and forced me out the door. He shoved my face with his hand, threw me on the grass, and pinned me down. I started punching, scratching, and kicking after I felt the blows to my face. Jamal had come out and broke us up.

"Man, y'all don't want to go to jail. They calling the cops on y'all."

I walked back to the hotel, which wasn't a long walk. I don't know where Raymond went.

"You want a ride back?" Jamal yelled.

I said nothing back. When I arrived, Jamal and a few others that went to the bar with us were telling the security guard what took place. He was an ATF agent working security at the hotel.

"Are you all right? Your friends were just telling me what happened. He's done this before, right? This isn't the first time. And he's going to do it again until you take a stand. Do you want to call an ambulance or press charges?"

"No."

"I tell you what, he cannot come back on this property, and if you're going to stay, I have to have you sign this."

*Perpetuality*

He was giving me the big brother talk as I signed the document, which stated Raymond was not to be allowed back on the property or he would be arrested.

"This guy has bruised your whole face. You call this love?"

I didn't realize my eye was black and blue. I felt bruised all over, that's for sure. My lips felt like water balloons. I had realized this was serious, being that Raymond was no longer allowed back on the premises, but at the same time, to me it was business as usual.

I went to my hotel room, which was on the third floor. When I got inside the room, I looked in the mirror. I looked a fucking mess. My right eye was black and blue, and my upper and lower lip was swollen. I was thanking God that none of my teeth got knocked out. My hair was out of place, and my clothes were muddy and dirty from fighting in the grass. I didn't know what to do with myself. I was so pissed, because I had a full plate of buffalo wings, fries, celery, and carrot sticks I had not eaten, and I was hungry. I had just asked for a doggy bag before I went to approach Raymond at the games. The phone started to ring. I thought, *Who the hell could this be calling me?*

"Hello?"

"Hey Boo Boo."

"Hey."

I was surprised to hear from him, especially so soon.

"I need you to look out for me. I'm laying on the floor in somebody's car. They're about to drive me in."

"What! Raymond, if you get caught you're going to jail."

"Listen, you know I don't have anywhere else to go. Just look out, okay? I should be up there in five minutes."

"Okay."

I don't think I realized at the time that I would be going down with him too, or I just ignored it and did what he said to. Yes, I ignored the facts, which was I-G-N-O-R-A-N-T. I stood by the door, constantly looking through the peephole and then back at the time on the alarm clock, palms and armpits sweaty. I don't know how he did it. I don't know where security was. It was about five minutes later that he got to the door.

"Lock the door. Make sure the curtains are closed all the way. I gotta piss," he whispered, trying not to be loud. The only light that was on was the one in the bathroom. He came out and laid on the bed with his jacket still on.

"Stupid-ass bitch. We wouldn't even be in this damn situation if it wasn't for you. So damn stupid. I can't stand your motherfucking ass."

I was sitting on the other side of the bed, facing the bathroom. My eyes got fixed on my shaver sitting on the counter. I don't know what came over me, but the next thing I knew, I had yanked him by his coat, and had the shaver to his throat.

"You know what, motherfucker? I am sick and tired of your ungrateful ass. Nigga, you see what you did to my face?"

"Boo, I'm sorry, calm the fuck down."

He couldn't get loud or do what he wanted to. He wasn't even supposed to be on the premises. The next couple of days, I would go to the store to get something to eat. I could tell he was starting to get antsy. One day when I got out of the shower, I thought I was tripping. Raymond wasn't in the room. I could've slapped myself for letting him back in.

"What the hell are you thinking, going out there? You're not even supposed to be on the property."

"Calm down. I called Jamal before I went up. Security isn't here right now. He said he'd be looking out. He got my back."

"Raymond, you don't know Jamal or anyone else around here. You really don't think people are watching you?"

*Perpetuality*

It got to the point a few other people knew he was back at the hotel.

One night we had just finished eating. We were relaxed, watching TV.

*Boom, boom, boom, boom, boom.* "Fulton County Police, open up!"

"Fuck!" Raymond said, trying to hide under the bed, but it wasn't working. There was nowhere to hide or run.

"I got bags of weed in the top drawer and in my jacket. Flush it down the toilet. Hurry up!" he whispered, trying to hide in the shower. Jamal had given him some dime bags to sell.

"Open the damn door. We know you're in there."

I thought I had lost control of my bladder and bowels. I opened the door.

"That's him," Zack told the officers.

"Listen Zack, I can explain."

"Shut the hell up. You have nothing to say."

When Zack the Security/ATF got the word that Raymond was back on the premises, he probably didn't want to believe it. I could just imagine him thinking, *I know she must have another man in here.*

I wished Raymond was somebody else, too. They forced Raymond face-down on the bed, and put him in handcuffs.

"You're under arrest for trespassing."

I got shoved against the wall, and was also handcuffed.

"Zack, I'm sorry man. I didn't have anywhere else to go."

The officers wanted to know where our IDs were. I told the lady officer it was in my purse, and then she put it in my pocket. The male officer got Raymond's ID out of the same drawer, where I had just removed the dime bags of weed and flushed it.

"Could ya'll please let my wife go? She can't go to jail."

"She should've thought about that before she let you back in."

"Zack, I will do anything, man. I got some information you would want to know. Can I talk to y'all outside please?"

Raymond had the gift of gab. Zack and the male officer took Raymond outside and put him in the cop car. The lady cop stayed with me in the room. I felt like I was having an out-of-body experience. About 15-20 minutes later, Zack, the male officer, and Raymond came back inside. Except, Raymond wasn't in handcuffs. The male cop motioned to Cindy, the lady cop, to take my handcuffs off.

"Y'all got until midnight to get your stuff and get out," Zack said, leaving through the door.

Whatever Raymond told them must have been good. I just knew I was going to be in a jail cell that night.

Raymond made a phone call to Oscar, Skye's husband. They had a house out in Stone Mountain. Mookie was her boyfriend on the side. Skye had taken us to her house to meet Oscar one day after she got off work at UPS.

Oscar was a mechanic. Raymond really wanted to meet Oscar after hearing that they had a lot in common. The same day they met, Raymond and Oscar clicked like twins. One of the things they did have in common is they both liked to drink, but Oscar was more laid back. Raymond and I had even encouraged Skye to go back to Oscar and try to make her marriage work. I remember the four of us having prayer together at their house. Going there was a last resort for us, because their house was a pig-sty, and there was the smell of mildew everywhere. Oscar went into a deep depression after Skye left. The only time she went to the house was to get clothes and check the mail.

Raymond had told Oscar what was going on and that we needed a place to stay.

"Thanks man. I appreciate it."

*Perpetuality*

Next thing I knew, Skye was at our door helping us take our luggage to her black Lincoln Navigator, which Oscar said he was paying the note on, and she had her boyfriend Mookie driving it sometimes. I was grateful that Skye and Oscar let us stay at their house.

Raymond had slapped Zack up on our way out.

"No hard feelings man?"

"No hard feelings. I hope you guys get it together. Get the hell out of here," Zack said with a smirk.

Raymond had explained in detail what had happened with us on our ride from Doraville to Stone Mountain.

Skye showed us to our room in back of the house.

"Hey, we ain't complaining," Raymond said.

"Sorry. Y'all will have to fix it up and everything. The frame for the bed should be in here somewhere."

There were bags of clothes and toys everywhere. Skye was in her mid-thirties with an 18-year-old daughter, and one or two grandchildren. It took us the whole night, until about six in the morning, to get the room tidy. Oscar and Skye agreed to let us stay until we got jobs and got on our feet.

I hadn't talked to my mom or any of my family in almost a month. I could feel my mother worrying about me. Oscar and Raymond had been gone for a minute. I had used the time to pray and worship. Suddenly, I heard a phone ringing. I was confused, because Oscar said that that their house phone wasn't in service. After it stopped ringing, I picked up the receiver, and there was a dial tone. I knew this was God working supernaturally.

"Thank you Jesus." I called my mom in an instant.

"Lana. Girl, we've all been worried about you. You've never gone this long without calling."

"I know, Mommy. I'm sorry. I am okay. We're staying with a couple of friends in Stone Mountain."

"I'm glad you called me. I thought we was going to have to report you missing."

"Oh, Raymond is coming in. I'll be in touch. I love you, Mommy."

"I love you too. Call me."

"I will."

There was a lot of food, including frozen meat that had not been touched. Skye never stayed around. She was still getting her groove on with Mookie, who was half her age. Oscar said he never cooked. He ate out a lot. Skye did all the cooking, but she had been gone for months. He told Raymond and I to help ourselves to anything in the kitchen. We ate breakfast, lunch, and dinner. We were cooking full course meals. One morning, I made pancakes, grits, sausage, bacon, eggs, and hash browns. Oscar and Raymond had already been drinking a 20 ounce of Bud Light. Raymond said it cured his hangover. Raymond got mad because I served Oscar his plate first.

"Stupid ass," Raymond mumbled. "How you gonna serve another man his food over me? I don't want that shit. I already lost my appetite."

I was flabbergasted. "I'm sorry. I didn't mean it like that."

"Raymond, you all right man? She didn't mean nothing by it."

Raymond left his plate of food on the table and went back to our room.

I'm thinking to myself, *Honestly, I hadn't meant any harm or disrespect*, because this man was letting us stay in his house rent-free and eating his food. I was just showing appreciation. I took my breakfast in the back where Raymond was. When I walked in the room, Raymond was facing the window.

"What the hell are you doing in here? Go and eat breakfast with your man. You probably want to suck his dick, too!"

I just ignored him and walked back to the dining area to finish my breakfast, because I was hungry. I put Raymond's plate in the microwave.

"Is he all right?" Oscar asked.

"I don't know what's wrong with him."

Oscar walked back to the room to talk to Raymond.

"Oscar, no offense man, but I don't even want to talk about it. That's my wife. I'm not mad at you, but she should know better."

"She didn't mean it like that, though."

Our room wasn't that far from the dining room. I could hear the conversation. Oscar came back from the room and went to go watch TV in the living room. After cleaning the dishes and the kitchen, I went back to our room where Raymond still was, to take a nap. I was so sleepy. Raymond was still facing the window when I laid next to him on the bed. As soon as I was about to drift off, here we go.

"I want a fucking divorce. How are you going to disrespect me like that? Then you really went back out there and ate breakfast with him? You didn't even bring my plate back here to see if I had changed my mind," he yelled, flaring his nostrils.

Raymond always was playing mind games. I just kept quiet with my back turned to him and didn't say anything. Raymond grabbed me by my shoulders and forced me on my back, then climbed on top of me, pulled his dick out of his boxers and said, "Suck my dick, dumb bitch."

"Stop, Raymond." I was squirming for him to get off me.

"You don't suck it right anyway. The other women I've been with suck dick way better than you do. You sound like a damn little girl. 'Stop, Raymond,'" he said mockingly.

He had pinned me down by the wrists and started licking my face like a beast or should I say demon. Then he spit on me and it went on my neck.

"Get off me!" I started to scream.

He put his hand over my nose and mouth. I tried biting his hand, but he took the pillow he was laying on and put it over my whole face. I was scratching and got room to scream really loud after I could catch a breath. I finally managed to get up, but he forced me in a corner, where he started beating the wall. Oscar rushed in the room and pulled Raymond back.

"Hey man, what the hell is wrong with you?"

Raymond got mad and began to get in Oscar's face.

"What you wanna do? That's my wife. You want to fuck her?"

"Yo, I'm not going to let you disrespect me in my own house. I don't even put my hands on Skye," he said as he walked away.

Raymond put on the rest of his clothes and walked out the front door.

"You know I'm going to have to ask him to leave, right?" Oscar said as he stood in the doorway.

"Yeah, I know. I am very sorry."

"I am too. You can stay, but he definitely got to go. Why are you putting up with that?"

All I could do is shake my head.

"That's a damn shame," Oscar said as he walked away.

I knew I wasn't going to stay there without Raymond. Later that afternoon, Skye showed up. Oscar had called her.

"I'm going to have to ask y'all to leave. I was trying to help y'all out. Lana, you can stay, but I know you're going to go with him." Skye looked pissed as she stood in the doorway. Oscar walked up beside her.

## Perpetuality

"I won't be disrespected in my own house. You're going to have to find somewhere else to stay. You burned your bridge here, bro."

"Oscar, you right man. I'm sorry y'all."

"We accept your apology, but you gotta find somewhere else ASAP," Skye stated. I could tell they were very disappointed as they walked away.

Raymond and I got on the phone to call his grandmother and my mother to buy our greyhound bus tickets for the next day. I didn't go into details with my mother, and he didn't go into details with his grandmother. We just told them both that we really needed to come home, because we weren't going to have a place to stay. Oscar and Skye were in the living room with us when we were making our reservations.

"Hey Oscar, and Skye, can we stay here until the morning? Our bus leaves tomorrow afternoon," Raymond asked them.

Oscar and Skye both agreed to let us stay until then. We told them thank you and went to the back room to start packing.

Skye and Oscar both showed us to the door that morning with our four to five bags of luggage. Scott gave us bus fair to get to the Greyhound station.

"Damn, they couldn't drop us off?" Raymond said as we walked to the bus stop.

I just shrugged my shoulders.

"We're going to be all right, Boo Boo," he said as he hugged me around my neck.

I just gave him a half smile. I didn't say much on the way to the bus station, or on our trip back to Rochester, New York, which took about a day or so.

We arrived back in the R.O.C. in the early evening. Mrs. Perry picked us up from the bus station downtown. Mrs. Perry gave a piece of her mind. She told Raymond he wasn't going to be able to stay long, because his grandfather was going to be on him. We stayed at his grandparents' house for about a week or so, and at his sister Carla's for about the same, until Raymond jumped on me and started choking me. Her boyfriend told him he had to go, and I went right behind him. We stayed from pillow to post. I had let myself go so bad. One afternoon, a family friend walked past me downtown while I waited for the bus. That's how unrecognizable I was.

His homeboy let us stay with him on Conkey Avenue. This was a drug-infested area. One night he left me there for hours. I remember seeing a big-ass rat on the stove, like he was looking for something to get into. I changed my mind about trying to make something to eat.

One morning, after a night when I hadn't slept much, a couple that stayed at the same house got into an altercation. The boyfriend had cut his girlfriend's arm and above her right eye with a knife. I told her she was going to need stitches. The ambulance was called. She lied and told them something else happened, not that her boyfriend tried to stab her. When the girlfriend left in the ambulance, Raymond and her boyfriend were laughing and joking about it. I was furious, and walked out the house. Raymond rushed up behind me and pushed me to the ground.

"Where you think your ass is going? You not going nowhere, bitch." I wanted to throw up from the way he looked as he shook me.

"Yo man, just let her go," one of his homeboys yelled.

It was a warm sunny day in summertime. Not only were his homeboys watching, but there were neighbors watching next door and across the street. I walked to the nearest bus stop to go to my mother Vanessa's house. I managed to pull myself together so she wouldn't keep asking me what was wrong. My mother felt better after I told her

*Perpetuality*

I was no longer going to be staying with Raymond on Conkey Avenue. She had picked me up a few times, and I could tell she was disgusted.

I started to focus on myself and did my best not to think about Raymond, who he was with, or what he was doing. I was working at a health care agency as a Certified Nursing Assistant. I was racking up on hours, taking any assignment and hours they gave me. Every time Raymond left a message for me to call him, I never called him back. I had made my own plans to find a job and move back to Atlanta.

When I arrived in Atlanta an early afternoon in March of 2005, I caught the Marta Bus to a motel on Wendell Drive, off of Fulton Industrial (not too much longer after I got there, the named changed to USA Economy Lodge). That same night I called my family to let them know I was safe, my brother Adam told me a Mr. Hickerson called about the C.N.A. position at The Renaissance on Peachtree.

"Really! He called today?" I squealed. That really made my night.

I called Mr. Hickerson first thing the next morning. He asked me if I had my CPR card and Georgia Nurse Aide Certification. I went in for the interview that same day. The interview was successful, and he hired me on the spot. I went to have my drug test done, which was within walking distance down the street. Talk about God's favor.

When I told him I didn't know my way around Atlanta too good, and that I couldn't afford to pay for the uniforms I needed, which was navy blue or white tops with kakis or navy blue pants, he offered to take me to a Walmart and he paid for it. I was so grateful. When he was dropping me off to the motel, he told me to be careful because it wasn't such a good area. And I knew it wasn't. The motel looked like a prison. The doors were painted black, and the room numbers were written really big in white paint. I thanked Mr. Hickerson for all his help, and told him I would see him the next Monday. I loved the fact that I didn't work weekends, just weekdays in the evening, 3-11 p.m.

About two weeks went by, and I couldn't get Raymond off my mind. My will power had run out. I called his mother and grandmother to tell them where I was. I asked them to have Raymond contact me as soon as they heard from him. In less than a week, he was knocking at the motel door. His friend Canon paid for his bus ticket. We hugged and kissed each other. We both agreed he needed to take a shower before we went any further. He was sweating bullets. He had a sweatshirt and sweatpants on. He didn't expect it to be so hot in Atlanta. After our honeymoon was over, I laid there with him knowing I had dug a deeper ditch for myself. He said he was going to start going to rehab at St. Joseph's in Midtown Atlanta. Never happened.

Along with a young black guy named Benny, Raymond and I got pulled over by the Atlanta Police Department at the gas station down the street from the motel. There were two cops that got out with their guns pointed at us in front. What was so tripped out was that Raymond had just let Benny take the wheel when they came out of the store with their snacks. I was in the passenger seat.

"Get out of the car slowly with both hands up. Now put them on top of the car."

As they walked toward us, 2-3 more cop cars showed up. As they patted us down, they said it was a stolen vehicle.

"Officer, someone let me borrow this car," Benny said.

I thought I was having a nightmare. I didn't know if I was coming or going. Before I knew it, I was handcuffed and put in the police car. All three of us were in separate police cars. Raymond was looking my way with a sorry look on his face. I started praying in my heavenly language to myself. I felt peace. It seemed like I was in the back of that police car for almost an hour or so. Benny told them that a white young crack fiend let him borrow the Grey Honda for a fix, and he'd asked if Raymond and I wanted to tag along. The crack fiend called

*Perpetuality*

the police because he got paranoid. The story checked out, and we were free to go.

# Chapter Eight

One morning Raymond suggested that we rent a car. We looked through the phonebook to get quotes from a few places. I reminded him I had to be at work at 3 p.m. that afternoon. We ended up going to Atlanta Rent-a-Car on Memorial Drive. I had just gotten paid, and had opened a new checking account at Bank of America and gotten a Georgia Driver's License. They rented to me a brown Ford Taurus. I let them see me get in the driver's seat and drive off so they wouldn't see me letting Raymond take the wheel, as he didn't have a license.

My confidence was really low when it came to driving. Raymond always cussed me out, called me stupid, and would say I didn't know how to drive. One time I was driving the red Plymouth Neon when we lived in Rochester, New York. He got so irritated and mad, he demanded I get out and get on the passenger's side at a red traffic light.

He dropped me off to work, even though I was running twenty minutes late. I had called ahead of time to let them know. We decided to try another hotel not too far away that looked a little better, called Inn Town Suites on Fulton Industrial. It cost a little more money, but it was better. It wasn't long before things got worse and worse.

It was about six o'clock in the morning, and someone was banging on the door. Nikko said I needed to come outside quickly, that it was about Raymond.

I could not believe what I was seeing. Raymond had blacked out. He was passed out face up on the concrete with the door opened, and the car was running. Only God knows how long he was out there before Nikko found him in the parking lot. He woke up cursing after we threw ice-cold water on him a few times.

*Perpetuality*

He would want to go out and drink at different clubs and strip joints right after I got out of work. I had no control of my finances. I was working full-time, and I got paid about $550 every two weeks.

One of my co-workers invited me to a barbeque for Memorial Day. She told me that I could bring Raymond. I was hesitant at first, but I agreed to come. Raymond and I stayed for a good while. We did have fun. We ate, danced, and mingled with folks. Then right at the end, it got bad. I couldn't quite hear what Raymond was asking this young lady. But she looked at him like he was crazy, and she was with a guy. I don't know if it was her boyfriend, husband, or what.

"Fuck you!" Raymond yelled out loud to the young woman.

"I am so sorry," I said, embarrassed. I could have crawled under a rock to hide myself. "Raymond, let's go. You have had too much to drink."

Come to find out the young lady was my co-worker's daughter-in-law. I apologized to her the next time I saw her at work.

We had started staying at the Aloha on Memorial Drive. He started talking me into stripping and getting into the escort business. I wore certain outfits to go audition at a few strip joints. After three or four auditions, I got hired at a strip club named Platinum 21. I had to go in the basement and strip butt-naked for the mother of the house.

"You got some pretty titties. Nice shape, too. What's your name?"

"Allana."

Where you from?"

"Rochester, New York."

"Oh yeah? I'm from Buffalo. You in, homegirl. You can start as soon as you get your permit."

The permit was $250. I was trying to figure out how I was going to get it. On the same Wednesday night, which was Platinum 21's amateur night, I decided to enter the stripping contest to win $500, even though I didn't have the outfit I wanted and my hair wasn't like I would have wanted it. It was just tapered down with Ampro gel. I kept telling Raymond no, and that I wasn't prepared, but he demanded that I do it, because we needed the money. He even forced me to give a lap dance before I got on stage.

"This your first time, ain't it? Don't be scared." The male customer smiled.

Before I knew it, I got a tap on the shoulder from another stripper. "House rules Ma, amateurs don't give lap dances," she said as she took over. I felt so out of pocket, especially after seeing Raymond suck his teeth and roll his eyes. I was ready to fucking go, but before I knew it, I heard my stage name being called.

"And now coming to the stage, Caramello!"

I was not present. Even though my body was there. I was just going through the motions. I was only given two minutes to show off what I had to Juvenile's song, "Back That Ass Up." I felt stiff as hell. My palms, underarms, and feet were sweaty. And a case of nausea kicked in. I have been told some dancers have to have a drink or two or do whatever before they hit the stage and work the pole. I understood it that night. I really did.

I don't know what the hell I was doing. I felt really low at this point. I had on a red bikini, with a red shimmering net blouse to cover, and black fashion sandals. I remember the DJ dissing my shoes, saying they looked like they were from the 1950's. I heard some boos and a couple of cheers from the crowd.

"Time's up Caramello. Y'all give her a hand," the DJ yelled. I looked and collected the dollar bills that were thrown at me. I got off stage and stood by Raymond in the back.

*Perpetuality*

"You did good, Boo Boo," Raymond said with a fake smile. I could always tell when he was lying buy the way his nostrils and his lips flared up at the same time.

"Thank you."

After the contest was over and the winner received her $500, Raymond and I went to the bar to get a drink. After a few minutes, Melody came over and told me I had done good, and that after I keep dancing and more practice, I would get used to it. Melody was one of the strippers we met when she gave Raymond and I a lap dance, about a week prior.

All of a sudden, gunshots rang out. People started screaming, ducking, and running.

"He's got a gun! He's got a gun!" a man yelled in the crowd.

Raymond grabbed me as I hit the floor. The suspect had gotten away.

"Let's go," Raymond said.

When we got in the car he asked, "Where's the money you got?"

I pulled it out my breasts and gave it to him.

"Thirteen, fourteen, fifteen. What the fuck are we supposed to do with fifteen dollars? Do you hear me talking to your stupid ass?"

I couldn't say shit. I was disappointed in myself that all I walked away with was $15.

A few nights back, we went to a handful of Kroger grocery stores to get about $600 cash back that I didn't have. My checking account ended up over $900 in the negative, with all of the bank fees included.

The next day, after the dance contest at Platinum 21, I paid to keep the Rent-a-Car longer. On several occasions Raymond would give different people a ride home after mingling with them at different clubs and after-hour parties we attended. Before the men would get out of the car, Raymond would tell me to show them my breast, and tell them to feel on them. They would give him the money. On one occasion, a black guy and woman followed us back to the Aloha Motel. Raymond told me to dance for them, and I did.

"She's real good. Got the body and everything. She could use some practice, which is not a problem."

I don't know what he and Raymond had discussed at the club prior to us coming back to the motel, but when he mentioned something about a contract, Raymond wasn't trying to hear it, and the guy left. The young woman stayed and taught me some moves and how to make it clap.

One morning after I got out of the shower, Raymond walked in with this man.

"Hey, Boo Boo. I want you to do a little something for him. He's going to give me some money when I give him a ride to where he has to go."

He directed the man where to sit on the floor, and he smoked his crack pipe while masturbating as he watched me play with myself butt-naked on the bed.

"Ten minutes, man. You got ten minutes," Raymond said as he left the room.

When the time came to give the fiend a ride, he said the person was not at home. Raymond left him where he stood, and only collected ten dollars.

"Raymond, we need to stop this. I can't do this anymore."

"Shut the fuck up, Lana. I'm trying to make us some money."

I had lost myself, but even more so, now I was being pimped. It got to the point we started living out of the rent-a-car. We were going to gas stations and laundromats to wash up. Raymond's cousin Linda came to Atlanta to visit her boyfriend in Stone Mountain one weekend. The four of us went to a club and had some drinks. At the end of the night, we drove around to see what parking lot or apartment complex we were going to sleep in. I remember one night having hot butt-naked sex in the car, the windows got really foggy, and we got approached by a security guard to keep it moving. The next couple of days, the smell of the car wasn't friendly at all. The mixture of dirty laundry, shrimp cocktail, liquor, weed, cigarette smoke, and sex. PADUSSY! Horrible smell, just horrible.

We were able to wash and dry our clothes at the house of a gentleman Raymond struck up a conversation with while we were ordering our food at Mrs. Winner's Chicken. His wife was nice enough to give me $5 when I asked for pads or tampons.

On one late night while we were eating at Waffle House, we met a guy that said he was a beautician, who Raymond started talking to. I made an appointment to get my hair done the next day before I went to work. Was this a beautician on crack? When I looked in the mirror, I looked like a confused twenty-year-old that was trying to be 80. Raymond cried out with extreme laughter. I was fucking pissed. I couldn't remember which was worse—this, or the time I tried to taper my hair in the back for the first time.

"What the fuck did you do, Lana? You look like you have a goddamn big-ass tea cup on your head!" Raymond said embarrassingly.

As soon as I got to work, I ran inside the nearest visitor's bathroom so I wouldn't be seen. I wet my hair in the sink and slicked it down with my Ampro Gel.

"Go, go, go! Shut up!" Raymond whispered.

Raymond walked behind me out of the store at the gas station. He had stolen a 20-ounce Bud Light and stuck it in my purse. He pulled in another gas station not too far away. When he came out of the store he looked pissed off. When he got in the car he said, "That goddamn

Arabian gonna tell me I had to pay twenty-five cents for some damn ice. I said ice this motherfucker, and threw it in his face."

"You did what?"

Speaking of gas stations, Raymond found a few Quick-Trips to fill the car up with gas, $25-$30 from time to time, and then sped off.

One morning we went to go seek help from World Conquerors International, where Crawford Doyle is Pastor in College Park. Raymond said he and Taneka had attended there when we were separated. They gave us a bag of groceries, a gas card, and we even got to see a marriage counselor for about an hour. She gave us a business card with our next appointment. That same night, Raymond pulled up to Magic City.

"What the hell are we doing here, Raymond?"

"Would you come on, I'm trying to have some fun," he said as he got out of the car.

"I don't fucking believe this," I whispered to myself.

I was able to sit at the table maybe about twenty minutes, and then I took the keys out of his jacket. I couldn't enjoy watching any strippers, let alone lap dances.

"I'll be outside until you finish."

"What! Where are you going?"

"I'll be in the car."

I'm sure the people passing by on their way in were wondering why I was sitting in the car.

I knew he didn't give a damn about us getting marriage counseling. The food and the gas card was good enough for him.

"How are you going to pull up at Magic City, after we just had marriage counseling hours ago?"

"Fuck it. We'll go somewhere else."

We pulled up at Bigelow's in Decatur, a club we use to go to with his cousins Mitch and Leah. The last time I remember going with them, I was praying to God not to throw up in the back seat of Mitch's Jaguar after drinking so much Hennessy and cranberry juice. Somehow I held it together.

Raymond got out of the car with his 16-ounce cup of beer. He was always drinking and driving. He turned back around when he realized I was still in the car.

"Get out the fucking car, Lana," he said as he walked up to the passenger side. I had the window rolled down nearly all the way.

"Splash."

Raymond took the 16-ounce cup of beer and threw it in my face. I was soaking wet, and the inside of the car was a mess. This guy was shaking his head as he passed by. "Now I got to go get another beer, messing around with your stupid ass," Raymond said when he got back in the car. When he pulled out of the parking lot, I started punching him all over and forgot about us being in traffic. He was trying to hold me back while driving. I called him just about every cuss word in the book.

"Don't you see these people looking at us?" Raymond yelled.

"I don't give a fuck!" I screamed back.

The gas station we pulled up to wasn't that far from Bigelow's, maybe a minute. When he got out of the car to go inside the store, I got in the driver's side to pull off. I drove down Gresham for almost ten minutes. I didn't know where I was going. I turned around and went back to the gas station where I left Raymond. When I pulled up, he was talking to a young guy behind the counter. It looked like Raymond said, "There she go."

"You know what, I'm not going to say shit to you, cause I'm going to end up killing your ass," he said when he got back in the car to drive. We finally found a parking lot to sleep in.

"I'm sorry, Boo Boo. You be making me mad sometimes. You still mad at me?"

All I could do is cry. I just remember feeling like shit and so tired. He let my seat back and began to give me oral sex. I wanted to bite his dick off when I was sucking it. He slapped me in the face and said, "Watch your damn teeth."

One day before I went to work, a guy he met at one of the clubs we attended let us take a shower at his house out in Sandy Springs. I don't know what happened, but when Raymond went to step out of the shower, he grabbed for the towel rack to hold on, missed, and fell flat on his face. *Splat!*

"Oh my God, Raymond, are you all right?" I asked, trying not to laugh.

"Yeah, I'm all right, just hurry up and get out of the shower." He was pissed.

"Y'all all right in there?" his homeboy shouted.

"Yeah, yeah," Raymond said as he walked out, laughing. I could hear him explaining what had happened. When we left his friend's house, Raymond told me to drive. I was waiting for him to give me directions after we got past a few lights.

"You don't know where the fuck you're going?" Raymond said with his hand on his head.

Raymond had just drunk a 211. Every time he drunk 211s, he was way over the top.

"Pull the fucking car over, Lana. Just pull over," he yelled, grabbing the wheel.

*Perpetuality*

When we got on the Georgia 400, Raymond went up to 100 mph, and it had just stopped raining.

"What the hell are you doing?"

"Don't you want to die together?"

I closed my eyes because I thought we were going to crash. He reared to the left to get off at the Peachtree exit.

When I got to work alive and with no broken bones, I walked pass Mr. Hickerson, as I went to go clock in.

"Hey Allana."

"Hello, Mr. Hickerson."

"You doing all right? Everything okay?" he said, very concerned.

"Yes, I'm okay," I replied hesitantly.

"I don't know about that. Let me know if you need to talk."

"Thank you, Mr. Hickerson."

I knew he was right. I wasn't the same person he had hired. My whole countenance had changed.

Mr. Hickerson found out I had a husband when Raymond showed up unannounced at my job and requested to see me at the front desk, where Mr. Hickerson would be sometimes with Annie, the receptionist. Annie was a seventy-year-old Italian woman who was a volunteer and looked as if she was fifty, and was sweet as can be. She also was a resident at the Renaissance. Then there was Victor, the security officer. Raymond came that day to get my bank card.

*Beep, beep, beep!* I received a page in the middle of dressing a client to call the front desk.

"Hey Allana, it's Victor. You have an emergency phone call about your mother in Rochester, New York."

"What!" I was frantic.

"Yeah, I'm about to connect you."

"Hey, Boo Boo."

"Raymond, security just told me there was an emergency with Mommy," I said, confused.

"Yeah. I told them that so you wouldn't get in trouble."

I had to remember I was at work and couldn't curse him out over the phone for telling this bold-faced lie.

"Listen, I found us a place to stay. I need to see you on your lunch break."

"Okay."

"Love you," he said, laughing.

"Love you, too."

I was so relieved that it wasn't an emergency phone call, but at the same time I was pissed off. My insides felt like they were in a blender, and I couldn't shut it off. My thoughts were everywhere. Thank God my break was coming up. Raymond knew I took my lunch break at 6:30 p.m.

"Don't you ever, I mean *ever*, lie about some shit like that again," I told him as he pulled in the parking space.

"I'm sorry. I was trying not to get you in trouble," he said while pulling out the newspaper.

"This is the place I called, Roslyn's Lodge. Only $110 a week," he said with a big smile. "I talked with Elizabeth, the manager, about not having a place to stay, and that you started your full-time job not too long ago, and that you will get paid on Friday. She said she will work with us, and she'll accept a personal check along with ID, and the office closes at 8 p.m. I told her you were at work." Raymond was getting so excited.

I was still trying to get over that phone call.

"Really? That's good," I said trying to sound excited. "You don't think Smyrna is too far?"

"Come on, Boo Boo, we have a place to stay."

"Yeah, that's true."

I was thinking about what it would feel like to finally take a nice hot shower as long as I wanted, and lay in a bed, which I hadn't done in a few months. Before I knew it, Raymond had already got my purse out the trunk.

"How you know I wanted you to get my purse?"

"Because you want to write this check," Raymond replied as we both laughed.

I exchanged the personal check and my driver's license for Elizabeth's phone number.

"I'll call her right away. Oh my God, I have to get back to work. It's almost 7:00," I said as I reached over to give Raymond a kiss.

He grabbed me gently by my head and stuck his tongue down my throat passionately. Then moved his tongue from side to side as if he was licking my other lips between my thighs.

"I'll finish the rest later. Love you."

"I love you, too."

As we were on our way to Smyrna, I prayed this wouldn't be a shabby hotel. I already was skeptical that we were even going to Cobb County, because of the racist rumors I heard about.

"Boo, you're going to really love it here. The room comes with a refrigerator and microwave."

"Really, a refrigerator and microwave?"

"Really. And the bed is king-size," he said with a smirk as he grabbed my thigh.

"Elizabeth seemed like a really nice lady when I talked to her over the phone."

"Yeah, she's really down to earth. Young, tall white lady. Looks like she's in her late 40s. She asked me, how long ya'll been married? I told her five years. She said, must be nice. She said you were so cute when I gave her your driver's license, and that you sure do have a handsome looking husband," he said as he blushed.

"And you liked that, didn't you?" I asked as I rolled my eyes.

"Don't get mad at me because Elizabeth want some of your big black dick," he said egotistically.

"Whatever."

As we pulled into Roslyn's Lodge, it was quiet and seemed isolated, in its own little world.

"We're on the second floor, Boo Boo, 218."

I fell back as soon as I sat on the bed.

"Ahhh! This feels so good."

"I can make you feel better," he said as he climbed on top of me and sucked on my neck.

"What do we have to eat?"

"Broccoli, carrots, mashed potatoes, baked chicken, rolls, and some fruit." I smiled as I opened the container.

I would always bring home food after work, because the kitchen would always hook us up—the C.N.A.s—after they finished serving the residents. A dictary aide would always call the floor to let us know when to come down to the kitchen. Raymond and I both had big appetites, and we still would have food leftover.

I was in the shower about ten minutes when Raymond walked in.

"Come on, Boo. I got a surprise for you."

I loved this part of Raymond, sweet and romantic. When I came out the bathroom, the lights and the TV were off. There were slow jams playing real low from the alarm clock.

"Come here, Boo Boo!"

Raymond was laying on the bed, naked, with a bath towel spread out next to him. I didn't realize how sore I was until Raymond started to massage me slowly and gently with baby oil and lotion, from head to toe.

"I don't want you to do nothing but relax," he said, licking my navel, and then proceeded to eat his dessert too.

\*\*\*

"Hurry up. Get on the driver's side."

"How are we going to do that when he already saw you, and he got that bright-ass light shining on us?" I said, pissed off.

"I know," Raymond responded shamefully as he held his head.

Raymond began to reach to put his seatbelt on, but he knew there was no use.

"Sir, do you know how fast you were going?"

"45, sir," Raymond replied.

"You were going 50 in a 40 mph zone. You're not wearing a seatbelt, either. I see you're driving a rental?"

"Yes, sir."

"I need to see the papers and your driver's license."

"I'm sorry Boo, I know I should start listening to you."

I just kept quiet and looked out the window with disgust. I had been getting on Raymond about his speeding and not wearing a seatbelt earlier that day.

"Okay. Who's Allana Wilson? Is that you, Ma'am?"

"Yes, sir."

"Let me see your driver's license."

I was starting to get more tense and nervous.

"Okay. Here's the deal. Raymond, you're coming with me tonight, because you're driving with a suspended license. Mrs. Wilson is free to go. Step out the vehicle nice and slow for me."

It seemed like I had been holding my breath forever. I crawled over to the driver's side and watched Raymond, through the side mirror, get handcuffed by the officer. The cop pulled up beside me.

"Raymond says to call his grandmother first thing in the morning."

*Thank God I remembered to get a calling card,* I thought to myself.

"Do you know how to get to the police station?"

"No, Sir."

"We're way down South Cobb, past the airport or base, you can't miss it."

"Thank you, Officer."

I don't know if anyone was watching what had just happened, it being a weekday after midnight. We got pulled over as soon as we were making our entrance into Roslyn's Lodge.

"Good morning Mrs. Perry," I said, taking a deep breath.

"Hey, Lana Bana. How are you doing? Where's Raymond?"

"Ugh. That's funny you asked that, because that's why I was calling. Raymond was arrested last night for driving without a license."

"That stupid motherfucker. Lord forgive me. I'd leave his stanking ass baby girl, if I was you, but that's your husband. How much is the bail?"

"Eight hundred dollars."

"Lord have mercy. When is he going to grow up and be a man?"

"I don't know."

"All right. I need to get dressed before I head to the store. You should be able to pick it up at Western Union by eleven."

"Thank you, Mrs. Perry."

"Uh huh. You're welcome."

Mrs. Perry was in her mid 60s, retired from Xerox where she had put in almost 30 years, with A1 credit, a house that was paid off, and she always had money saved.

*Perpetuality*

"Okay Ma'am, I just need you to sign this paperwork for me. Here's your receipt, and this is Raymond's court date," the Officer said after counting the $800 in cash, looking like he couldn't believe it. I believe he was surprised that Raymond and I were a young black couple and that the bail was posted so soon.

"Are you waiting for him to come out?"

"Yes, sir."

"All right. You can have a seat around the corner here. He's got to get processed, so it should be no longer than an hour."

"Thank you."

I was surprised because it was small and quiet. A very calm atmosphere to be called a jail.

"Hey Boo Boo," Raymond said, cheesing as he made his way to give me a kiss.

"You miss me?"

"Yes," I said with a blush.

"Y'all be safe." The officer said at the counter as we walked out.

"Thanks," Raymond said, looking like he was glad to get out of there.

"You all right?"

"Yeah. I wasn't in there long, and they fed me good, too. My momma always come through for me. Thank you too, Boo Boo," he said, bragging. "I got court on the 29th of August."

"I see."

"You're going to have to remind me," he said as he grabbed my waist.

I sure did miss having that rent-a-car, but not for my freedom. Atlanta Rent-a-Car kept calling Mrs. Perry because I used her for a reference. They were going to put out a warrant because the car was in my possession past the turn-in date.

Coming from Smyrna took about 2 ½-3 hours. I would leave about 11:00am from Roslyn's Lodge to make it to work at 3pm. Having to catch three buses from Cobb County to the Arts Center Station in Atlanta, and then ride a Marta Bus to work was tedious and time-consuming. The commute took even longer at night. I took the bus from Brookhaven Station since it didn't take long, about five minutes, then take the Marta Train back to Arts Center Station to catch the Cobb County Transit Bus (CCT), the #10, to the Marietta Transfer Center, then ride the CCT #40 to Lake and Pine. I couldn't catch the last bus that left that intersection to take me to Roslyn's Lodge, because the last bus stopped running at 9:00 p.m. I was already leaving work early at 10:00 p.m. to make the last CCT #40, which left at 11:30 p.m.

The walk to Roslyn's Lodge was a good thirty minutes. Raymond would meet me at the Waffle House on the corner across from the cemetery, but some nights he didn't show up.

"Oh my God! What's wrong, Boo?"

"I don't know. I can't walk anymore," I said, bending over in pain.

It felt like somebody was putting their hand in my abdomen and squeezing it. Somehow Raymond managed to help me, almost carrying me across the street to the gas station to see if we could hitch a ride.

"Ma'am, I'm sorry to bother you. My wife isn't feeling well. Would you be able to give us a ride down the street to Roslyn's Lodge?" Raymond asked with a pitiful look.

The Caucasian lady looked over at me while pumping her gas.

"Sure. If ya'll don't mind riding with Buster."

Buster was her German Shepard that looked like he took up the whole car. She directed Buster to the passenger seat, and had Raymond and I sit in the back.

"My name is Raymond, and this is my wife Allana."

"Nice to meet y'all. My name is Kathy and this is Buster." She said with a giggle.

"Thank you very much for the ride. I don't know what happened. We were walking, and all of a sudden I got this excruciating pain.

"I know how that is," said Karen.

What was so odd was, it wasn't time for my period, and this didn't feel like my regular cramps. This pain was on a whole other level.

"Lay down and get some rest, Boo Boo. I'll be back in a little bit."

We hadn't been at Roslyn's Lodge long, maybe almost three weeks, and Raymond was already mingling with the neighbors, the folk he could drink with. I was so glad it was the weekend, and the next day was Saturday, because the CCT buses didn't operate on Sundays. I had already made up my mind to go to Piedmont Hospital to see what was going on with me, even though I didn't have health insurance. I didn't care about the bill.

After I saw triage and sat back in the lobby waiting to be called, I thought about how Raymond didn't come in until 5:30 that morning. I felt alone, and was very hurt that he hadn't offered to come with me to the hospital. It gave me flashbacks to about four years prior, when I was diagnosed with the Human Papilloma Virus (HPV), and I had to have a colposcopy, a cervical biopsy, and my doctor also gave me a Hysterosalpingogram (HSG) to make sure I was able to get pregnant. Around that time, my period was really late, thirty days or more. I thought I was having morning sickness because I suddenly had started vomiting after 6 a.m. as I was getting ready for work, and I had to call in. Raymond never knew that I had taken two home pregnancy tests, because one part of me wanted to surprise him with a positive test in a gift box, but they were both negative. Sometimes I wonder if I had a miscarriage without even knowing it. Did I ignore the clots in my blood and shrug it off as just a bad period due to stress?

Raymond never showed up for the Colposcopy Exam. Thank God I had swallowed my pride. Mommy and Aunt Charmaine both showed up, and were there until the end to take me home.

"Well, Mrs. Wilson, your pregnancy test came back negative. You don't have any Sexually Transmitted Diseases (STDs), but you do have a Urinary Tract Infection (UTI). I'm going to write you a prescription for an antibiotic and then you're good to go. Make sure you take all the medication," Nurse Betty insisted.

"Thank you."

"You're very welcome. Do you have any questions or concerns?"

"Yes. Why do you tell me to take all the medication?"

"Well, in order for the UTI to be fully treated, all the medication must be taken."

"Oh. I see. Thank you. Enjoy the rest of your weekend."

*** 

*Pop, pop pop pop pop pop pop pop!*

"Aaaaaaah! Lana!" Raymond yelled.

I was getting out of the shower.

"What's wrong? Oh my God!"

"I'm burning, I'm burning," he said in pain.

There were egg yolks and eggshells splattered all over Raymond and the room. It was a mess.

"911, what's your emergency?"

"Yes, I need an ambulance right away to 5950 Roslyn Drive, my husband has been burned, and he's in a lot of pain."

"Okay Ma'am, what's your husband's name and how old is he?"

*Perpetuality*

"Raymond Wilson, and he's twenty-eight."
"Are you his wife?"
"Yes."
"What's your name?"
"Allana Wilson."
I was starting to get very irritated.
"Is he conscious? Is he breathing?"
"Yes."
"Okay. Tell me, how was he burned?"
"He tried to cook about six or seven eggs in the microwave and then they exploded."
"Okay. I want you to keep some cold towels on him. The ambulance is on their way."

The ambulance took forever and a day. Then on the way to Austell Hospital, it seemed like they were driving 20 mph.

"Oh my fucking god. Ya'll is the slowest people I ever saw in my life. What the hell is taking so long? Ain't no damn traffic," Raymond yelled in frustration.

This was not the time to say *I told you so*, but all I could think about is when I told him there was no way for us to cook the eggs and I didn't think it would be safe to cook them in the microwave, but he insisted. After all, what the hell did I know? I didn't know a damn thing. I was just a stupid ass, Raymond told me.

\* \* \*

"Who is it?" Dalvin replied, looking through the peephole.
"It's Officer Kemp. I need to ask you a few questions, please."
I just knew we were busted. I knew without a shadow of a doubt they had found us, and we were going down. Raymond and I were

laying on our backs, side by side on the floor behind the couch, about eight feet from where Officer Kemp was standing in the door, shining his bright flashlight inside.

"*You have a collect call from Allana at Fulton County Corrections. To accept press one, to decline press 2.*"

"Hello?"

"Hey, Mommy."

"Oh my God Lana, what the hell is going on? Why are you in jail? Where's Raymond?"

All I could do is imagine what it was going to be like having to make that phone call to my mother.

"Hi, I'm officer Kemp. Sorry to bother you. What's your name?"

"Dalvin."

"Dalvin, do you live by yourself?"

"No, Sir. I have two roommates. They're still sleeping."

"Dalvin, have you heard any disturbing noises?"

"No Sir. I haven't heard anything. Everything okay?"

"We're looking for a man and a woman, both Black. We got a call they were breaking and entering."

"Wow. I hope you find them."

"Thank you for your time."

Dalvin could have given us up, but God.

This all went down about five o'clock in the morning, after Raymond and I got dropped off by a stranger, a white bald guy named Jimmy in his late fifties who we met at a bar in Chamblee. Raymond wanted to stay until it closed at four o'clock, and while there he blatantly disrespected me, flirting with another woman while they played pool together. He was bragging how good he was with his stick, and how he could show her better than he could tell her. Jimmy let us ride in the back of his red pickup truck. I remember Raymond looking at me with an evil, demonic look.

"Who the hell do you think you are?"

"I should throw your ass out the back of this truck."

He got mad because I checked him about flirting with the woman he was playing pool with. Jimmy dropped us off at Plantation Creek on Roswell Road. Dalvin had let us into his place after being awakened by Raymond harassing Pico and his brother Phillip to let us in their apartment, which was upstairs from Dalvin. Raymond and I had been sleeping on their floor, and in the vacant apartment next door that had been left unlocked for about two weeks, until we got approved for our apartment. After Raymond banged, yelled, and even kicked the door with the Timberland boots he was wearing, we realized Pico and Phillip weren't going to let us in. We went to the vacant apartment next door, only this time, the door was locked. Raymond attempted to climb through the window, and I was right behind him.

"Get out! Out!" a lady screamed.

"Oh shit! Fuck!"

All I know is, when we ran downstairs trying to escape, Dalvin was standing in the doorway trying to see what was going on, and let us come inside. Dalvin was another one of Raymond's drinking buddies that he got acquainted with that week.

After the police left, I woke a few hours later, about 8 a.m. The sun was beaming. I remember thinking to myself, *Was last night a dream?* I was in awe at the same time that I hadn't been arrested and put behind bars. In the same moment, I had to overcome the paralyzed fear to get up and leave. As I laid on the floor beside Raymond, who was hung over, I knew that I had come to a crossroad. I thought about the refund check of $850 he had in his pocket, that he had taken control over, that was in both our names. I had the unction to get up and leave before he woke up. I didn't use the bathroom, wash up, or anything. I took some soap, toiletries, and another uniform for work. I had made up my mind that I'd freshen up at work before my shift started.

"You want something to drink?" Dalvin asked.

"No, thank you. I have to get to work. Thanks for all your help."

I didn't stick around to have conversation about anything. The walk from Dalvin's apartment to the bus stop was a good fifteen minutes. I was praying that I wouldn't be stopped by Raymond. I had even thought about the possibility of being watched by the police. I kept looking over my shoulder, walking on pins and needles, trying not to seem too obvious at the same time.

Thank you, Jesus. I made it to the bus stop. It seemed like it took forever for the bus to come. I was finally able to exhale when I got on the #87.

As I approached the walkway to go inside my job, I heard my name being called.

"Lana!" Raymond yelled as he got out of the passenger side of the black rusty Honda. "Why did you just get up and leave?"

I could tell he had just woken up.

"Raymond, you were knocked out cold. I had to make a stop before I went to work."

"Whatever. Why'd you take the check?"

"I don't have the check. You had it."

"You didn't take the refund check?" he said with a confused and disgusted look on his face.

"Damn."

He just turned away and walked back to the car. I didn't know who the young white guy was who gave him a ride. I didn't hear *baby I'm sorry*, or *are you okay*. He left me standing there dumbfounded.

*Perpetuality*

Later that evening, about 7:30 p.m., I was helping one of my residents into bed, and noticed Bishop T.D Jakes on TV. The name of the message was "Suicide Watch". What caught my attention is when he gave the analogy about a fire coming towards you from behind and killing you, vs. you risking breaking a couple of bones if you jump; then, at least you would have survived. I knew that message was divine. The Holy Spirit was speaking to me. I didn't want to die, so I had to make a decision to survive. I called United Way 311 for Atlanta. I told them I couldn't go back to my husband, and I needed a place to stay. They connected me to the National Domestic Violence Hotline (NDVH), 1-800-799-7233. I knew when I made the call I was making the right decision.

"Thank you for calling the National Domestic Violence Hotline, this is Sara, and may I ask your name please?"

"Allana Wilson."

"Hi, Allana. Thank you for calling. Allana, are you in a safe place right now?"

"Yes. I'm at work right now."

"Okay, great. Allana, I just need to ask you some questions about you and your partner. Are you all right with that?"

"Yes, I am."

"Thank you Allana. What is your partner's name?"

"Raymond Wilson."

"And how old is Raymond?"

"27."

"How long have you been in a relationship with Raymond?"

"Nine years."

"Okay. Are you boyfriend and girlfriend?"

"He's my husband."

"Can you explain what's been occurring up until now?"

"Well, he's very controlling," I said hesitantly.

"Allana, has he ever called you names, pushed, kicked, or hit you in any way?"

"Yes."

"Has it gotten worse?"

"Yes."

"Allana, I commend you for taking a stand and making the call, because unfortunately this isn't going to get any better, especially if Raymond doesn't get any help. I want to let you know you're making the right decision. Allana, are you able to hold on for a few minutes please?"

"Yes, I am."

Sara was very encouraging, and I could feel her sincerity over the phone.

"Allana, are you still there?"

"Yes."

"Allana, I'm going to connect you to Lanette at Partners Against Domestic Violence (PADV) in Atlanta. I wish you all the best."

"Thank you," I said, thinking to myself, *Wow, this is serious.*

"You're very welcome."

"Hi Allana, this is Lanette from PADV. Where do you work?"

"The Renaissance on Peachtree."

"And where is that located?"

"On Peachtree Road."

"Allana, are you driving?"

"No, I am on the Marta."

"And what time do you get off work?"

"10:00 p.m."

"Allana, will you be able to take the train to North Avenue Station?"

*Perpetuality*

"Yes. I can do that."

"Good. I want you to call me at this toll-free number, 1-800-799-7233, when you arrive at North Avenue Station, and again my name is Lanette."

"Thank you, Lanette."

It was about 11:00 p.m. when I arrived at North Avenue Station. I called Lanette as soon as I could find a pay phone. She asked me to give her a brief description of what I was wearing so that the Fulton County Police Officer, who was coming to pick me up, could identify who I was. It made me remember a conversation my mom and I had about her having to get a life insurance policy on me, because she thought I would end up dead and she would have to identify my body.

The police officer was going to escort me to the women's shelter. It wasn't long before he arrived, maybe fifteen minutes.

"What is your name, Ma'am?"

"Allana Wilson," I stated.

He told me to get in the back seat. This whole transition felt weird and scary, but I knew I had to keep moving forward. "I'm Officer Bentley, and I'll be taking you to the women's shelter."

I felt safe with Officer Bentley. He was white, in his late 40s maybe, and had the voice of Teddy Pendergrass. How funny is that?

Lanette directed me to the room I was going to be staying in after she did my intake, which took about an hour. The intake involved numerous questions that asked details about Raymond and me, and the history of our relationship.

There were three other women in the room. My bed was all ready for me on the top bunk. I didn't have to worry about where I was going to store any luggage or bags. I brought only myself and the clothes on my back.

I can't explain the peace I felt when I woke up that afternoon. I had slept over ten hours. It was going on twelve o'clock in the afternoon, and I was the only one in the room. It was a bright Saturday afternoon. I felt so good. My body felt so relaxed and rested. I couldn't remember the last time I had felt so much peace and safety. I was able to get something to wear from the clothes closet, and Lanette had given me some toiletries, pads, tampons, and washcloths when I came in Friday night. All of my needs were being met.

I had an appointment to meet with my caseworker Jennifer that Monday at 10:30 a.m. I had appreciated Lanette scheduling me early, being that it was on a Monday, and I had to be to work at 3 p.m. Lanette had made my appointment during my intake Friday night. The reality of how serious my situation was started to kick in when Jennifer told me I had to resign from my job at The Renaissance on Peachtree. It was for my safety, and the safety of the other women at the shelter, because Raymond knew where I worked. He could follow me from my job to the women's shelter without me even knowing it. Jennifer asked me what my plan was regarding my relationship with Raymond. I told her my plan was to divorce him.

* * *

"Are you all right?" Mr. Hickerson asked.

I let a few tears flow.

"It's going to be all right, Allana. You're going to be all right."

I was so embarrassed and hurt. I had apologized to Mr. Hickerson and Sue the nurse for having to resign on such short notice. I showed them the letter from my caseworker for proof. Sue and Mr. Hickerson were very supportive of me. They told me not to worry, and were just glad I was okay and safe. I was able to use them for future job references.

"Call me if you need anything," Mr. Hickerson said as he hugged me.

"Thank you for everything."

It took everything I had in me to hold it together. I was starting to get choked up. Thank God the restroom wasn't far when I got off the elevator. I ran the water and flushed the toilet so no one could hear me crying. I was so devastated and broken. But in the midst of my brokenness, I had to move forward.

In less than two months of me being at the women's shelter, I started a new full-time job with more pay and good benefits at Emory Crawford Long Hospital, which was in walking distance in the heart of Midtown. I was able to file for my divorce for free. God was working everything out for my good. Hallelujah! On the 60th day from the time I filed, I was no longer married to Raymond Wilson. I didn't know whether to shout, scream, dance, skip, or jump when I heard the judge hit the gavel.

"Your divorce is final. Have a good day, Ms. Wilson."

*Allana Davis*

# YOU'RE THE BEAUTIFUL WOMAN GOD CREATED YOU TO BE

No matter how big or small, skinny or tall, You are the beautiful woman God created you to be. No matter how you feel, happy or sad, mad or glad, You are the beautiful woman God created you to be. No matter what people say or think, how many obstacles get in your way, You are the beautiful woman God created you to be. So hold your head up high and be strong. In spite of your flaws and all your wrongs, just remember, you are the beautiful woman God created you to be.

National Domestic Violence Hotline: 1-800-799-7233

Maybe you are still in denial or disbelief, or still doubting yourself. STOP IT! H.E.E.D. THE RED FLAGS! (HATE+ ENVY + ENMITY + DENIAL & DISORIENTATION = DEATH)

## Chapter Nine

Woman, if you don't get anything else from reading this book, remember: DO NOT TELL your abuser that you're going to leave, or anyone **YOU AND YOUR ABUSER ARE AFFILIATED WITH**, not even your mother. It may be hard, but do not utter a word to someone you can really trust until you make it to a safe place. Act as if you're planning a surprise birthday party for the one you love, except that you're planning your getaway to save your life.

Whenever you get to be alone by yourself, call **THE NATIONAL DOMESTIC VIOLENCE HOTLINE: 1-800-799-7233,** and if you know for sure your abuser is not monitoring your computer usage, you can get help at **thehotline.org**.

If you are working, please make arrangements to resign from your job after you have left your abuser. Don't take it lightly that your abuser may try to attack or kill you. More than likely, your abuser's ego will be crushed because you have finally gotten the courage to leave. You must stop going to all the familiar places your abuser knows about, including your job, church, school, babysitter if you have children, etc.

Have you ever heard the sayings, "When you find your head in the mouth of a lion, remove it slowly", and "Never let your right hand know what your left hand is doing"? In other words, if you're in a situation where you just happen to be with a mentally ill person, and you're concerned or afraid of how shit will go down, don't let them know anything you are planning or doing. You have to be strategic and come up with a plan, even if that plan is to not return home after work. Just don't return back to that job or any familiar places.

You can always replace material things and paperwork, but you CANNOT REPLACE YOUR LIFE! Trust the God in you. You can do it. I believe in you. Believe in yourself. It's okay to not have all the answers, and to be afraid of the unknown. Ask God for his help, and he will guide you.

Try your best not to panic or show frustration; it will give your abuser a heads up that something is going on with you or that you're up to something. BE AS STRATEGIC AS YOU CAN UPON YOUR EXIT! Get the mind of a WARRIOR, asking God for his divine wisdom. Expect some opposition—for example, your abuser may turn nice, wanting to do right all of a sudden, romance you back into the web of their control. It's okay. Go along with it to a degree, but STAY FOCUSED ON YOUR TASK!

Think of it as if you have booby traps here and there, laid out before you, and you have to be careful where you land your feet, but you still have to move, you have to get to the other side. PART OF HAVING A STRATEGY IS BEING TACTICAL! You already have the upper hand on your opponent (abuser), because you already have learned their ways and behavior. This is not the time to doubt who they are, or to start doubting yourself. Especially when they have showed their ass over and over again.

DO NOT BE DECEIVED, GOD IS NOT MOCKED! Woman, if you are married to a so-called pastor, bishop, apostle, prophet, or whatever title—doctor lawyer, police officer, whatever—and he is abusing you in any way, REMOVE YOURSELF! That is not a man of God you are submitting to.

Stop submitting to those demons. Be honest with yourself and to thyself be true. You are a spiritual being, and the God in you is helping you. This is where you put your faith into action and forgive yourself. You are strong, you are courageous, and you are victorious.

# Acknowledgments

To my husband, my chocolate drop and God's gift to me, Kenneth Davis Sr., I am grateful—and thank you for dealing with me and accepting my silent scars, my highs and lows. I love you so much. I am grateful and thankful for my mommy, Shirlene Little, my daddy, the late Allen Howard Parrish Sr., and my grandma, Annie Pearl Jackson, and to my sisters and brothers, Aleatha, Alesia, Allen Jr., and Alvin Parrish. I love you all so much. Thank you for always being there and for never giving up on me.

www.ingramcontent.com/pod-product-compliance
Lightning Source LLC
Chambersburg PA
CBHW070302010526
44108CB00039B/1644